Getting Ready for My Bone Surgery

A Broken Bone Recovery Guide for Kids

This book belongs to:

___

Written by Dr. Fei Zheng-Ward   Illustrated by Moch. Fajar Shobaru

Copyright © 2025 Fei Zheng-Ward

All rights reserved. Published by Fei Zheng-Ward, an imprint of FZWbooks. No part of this book may be copied, reproduced, recorded, transmitted, or stored by any means or in any form, electronic or mechanical, without obtaining prior written permission from the copyright owner.

Identifiers: ISBN 979-8-89318-134-0 (eBook)
              ISBN 979-8-89318-135-7 (paperback)
              ISBN 979-8-89318-136-4 (hardcover)

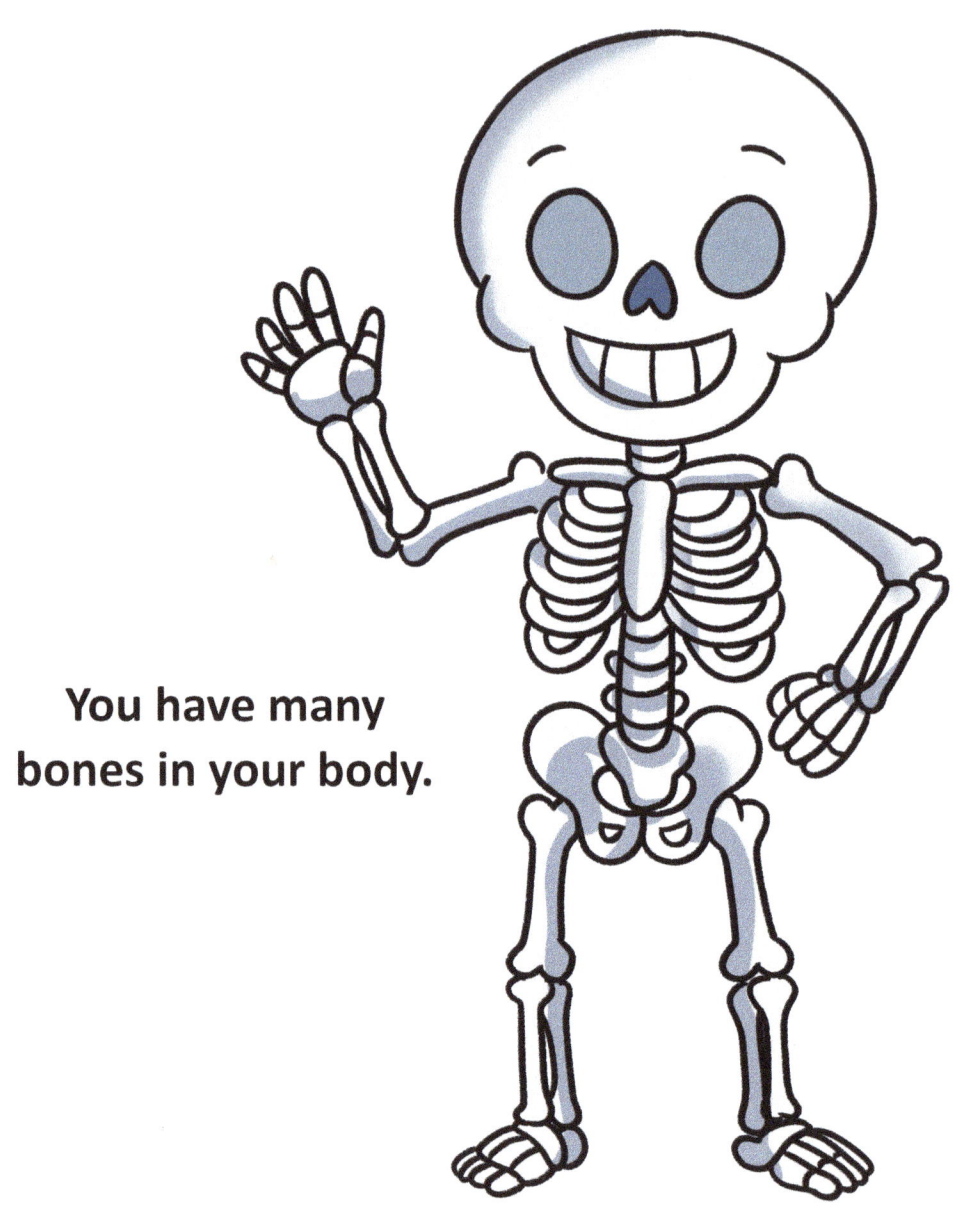

You have many bones in your body.

Can you guess how many bones you have? Circle your answer below.

10   50   100   more than 200

Your bones hold you up and help you sit, walk, run, and jump.

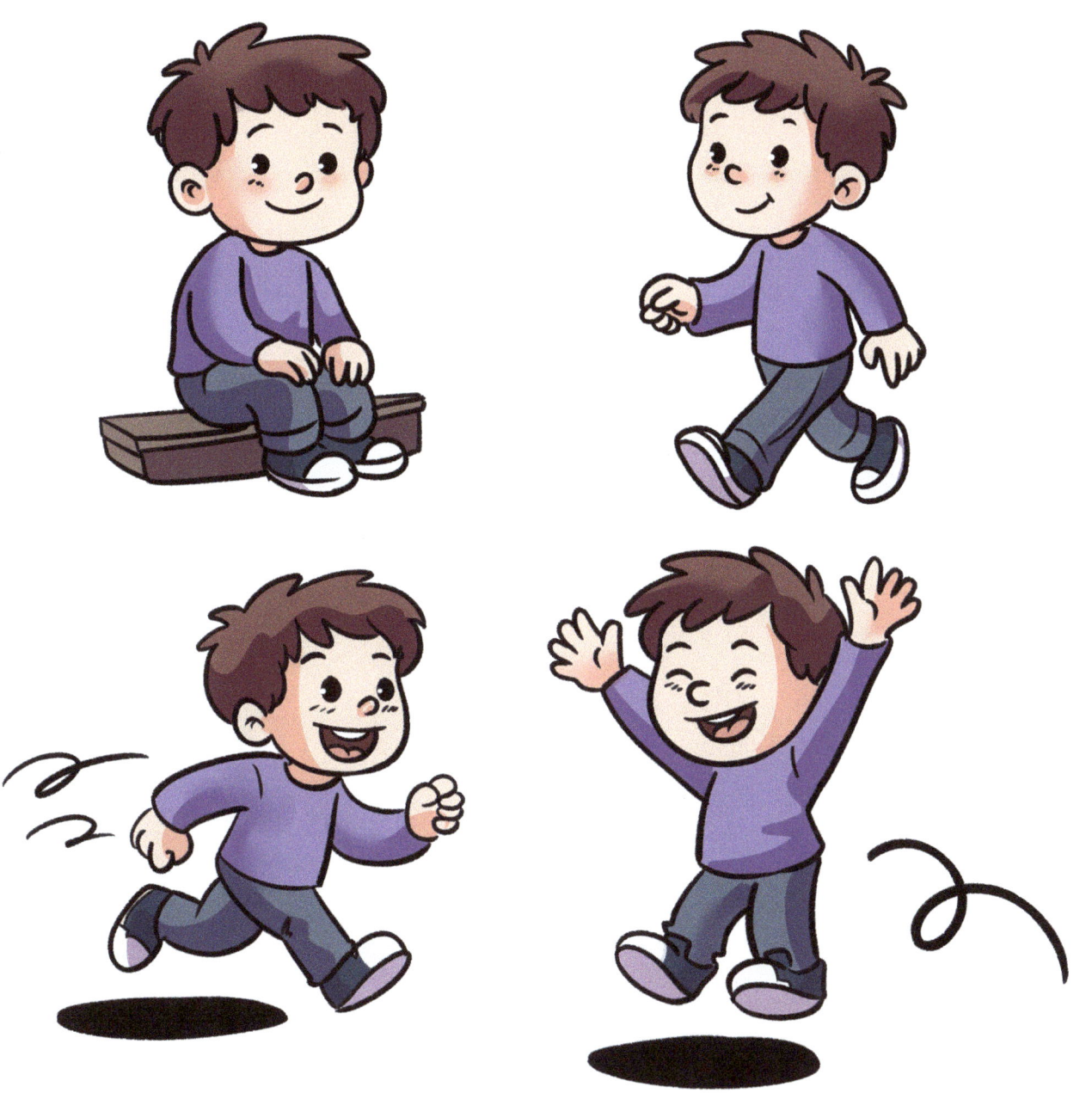

Answer: more than 200

Even though bones are strong, they can sometimes break.

When a bone breaks, it is called a fracture.
A fracture means the bone has a crack or is broken.

To see your fracture, your doctor often takes an X-ray picture.
An X-ray is like a special camera that lets your doctor look inside your body and see the broken bone clearly.

Don't worry—X-ray pictures don't hurt at all!

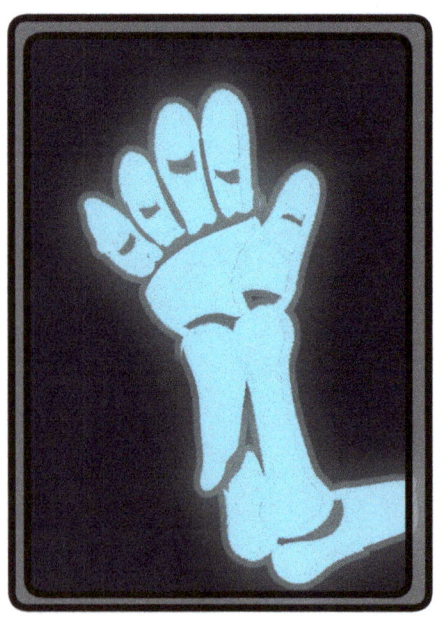 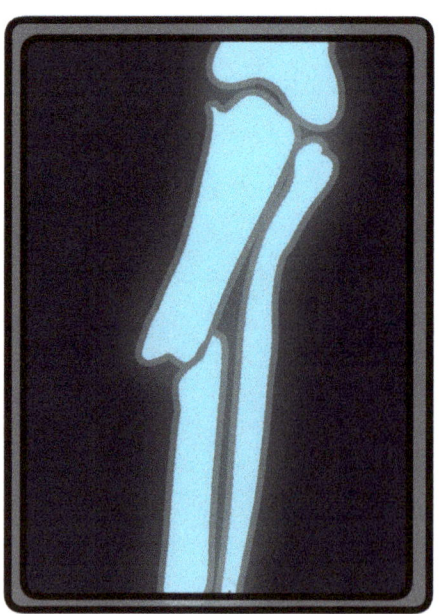

Can you spot the fractures in the pictures?

How did you break your bone?

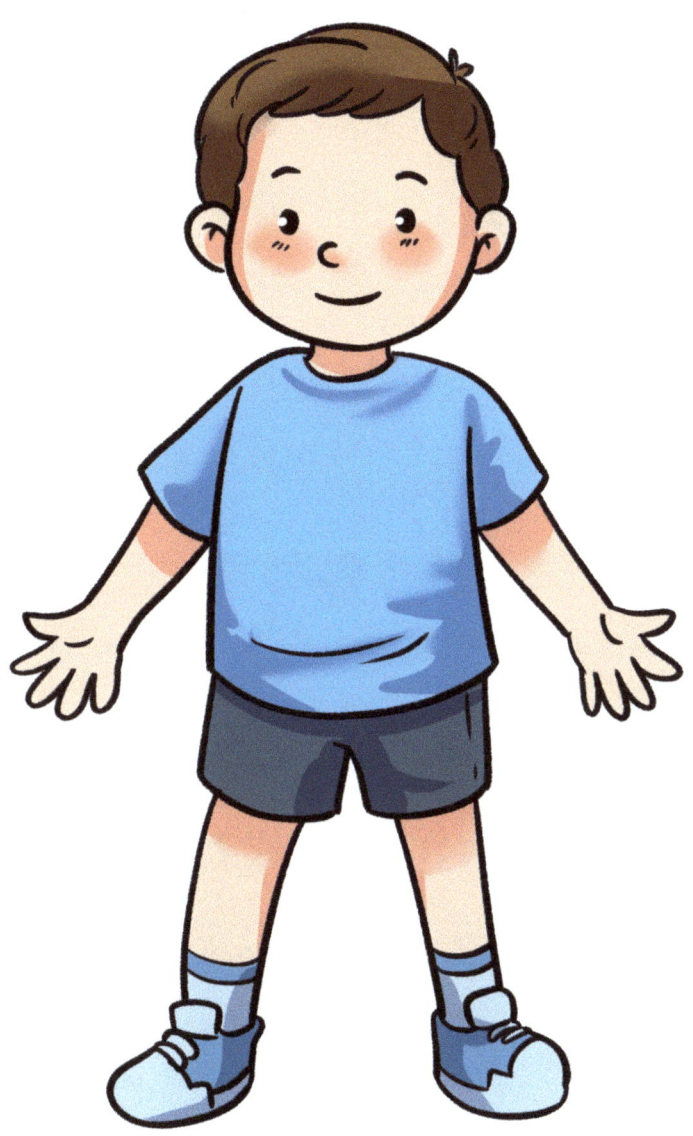

Circle the part of the body where your broken bone is located.

Sometimes, broken bones heal on their own.
Other times, your doctor needs to fix them with surgery.

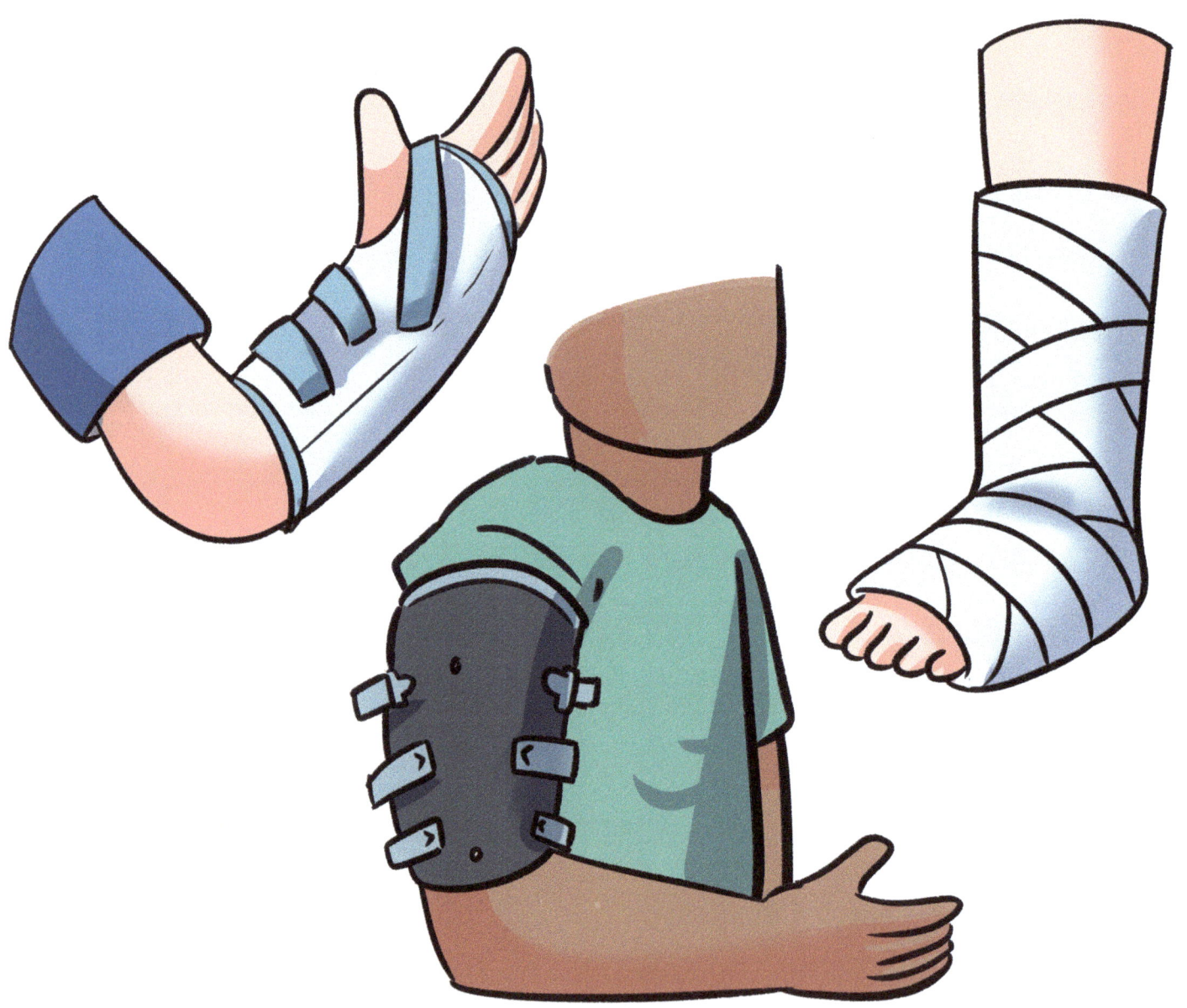

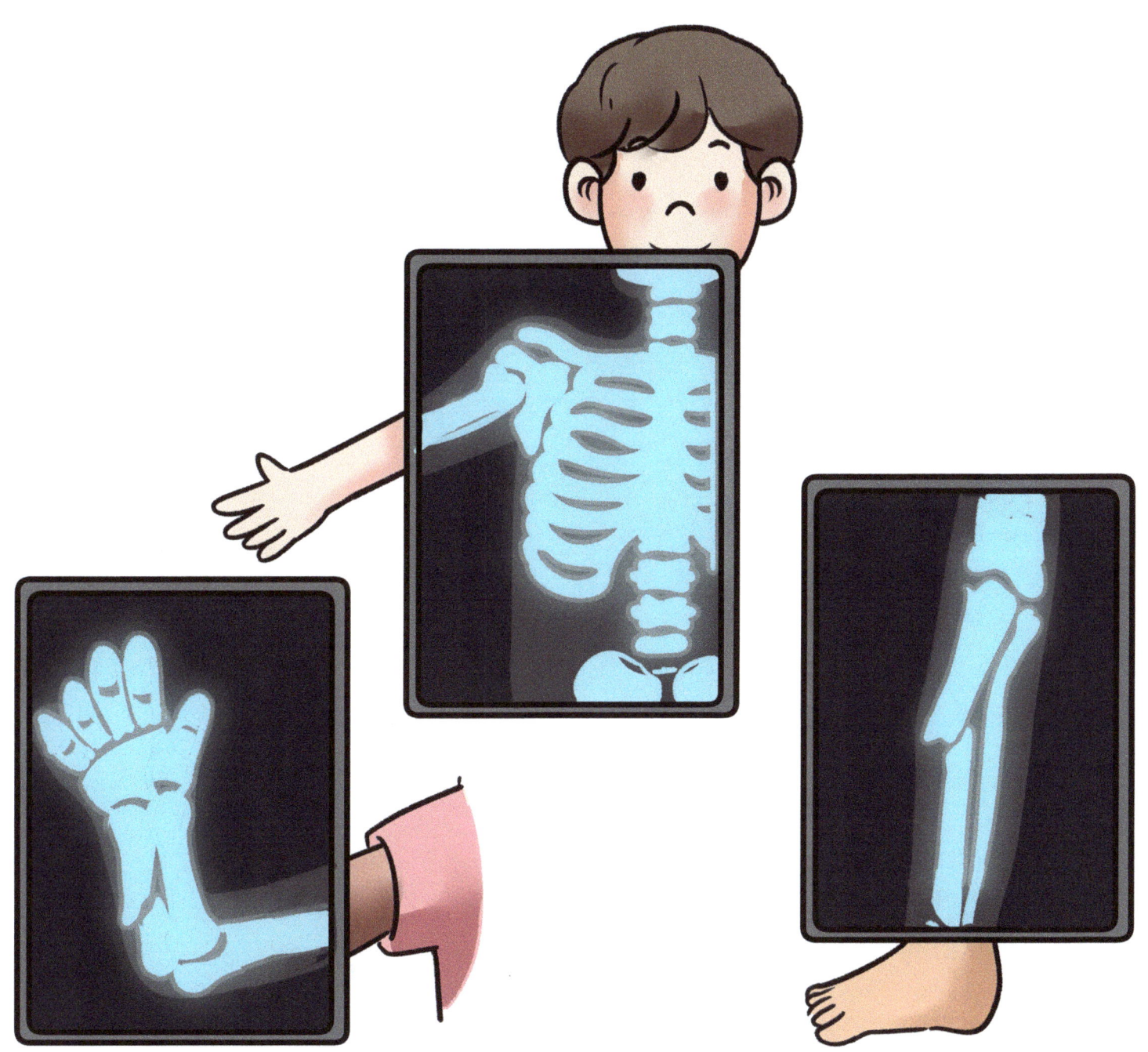

Your X-ray pictures help your doctor see exactly what's going on and decide what kind of care you need.

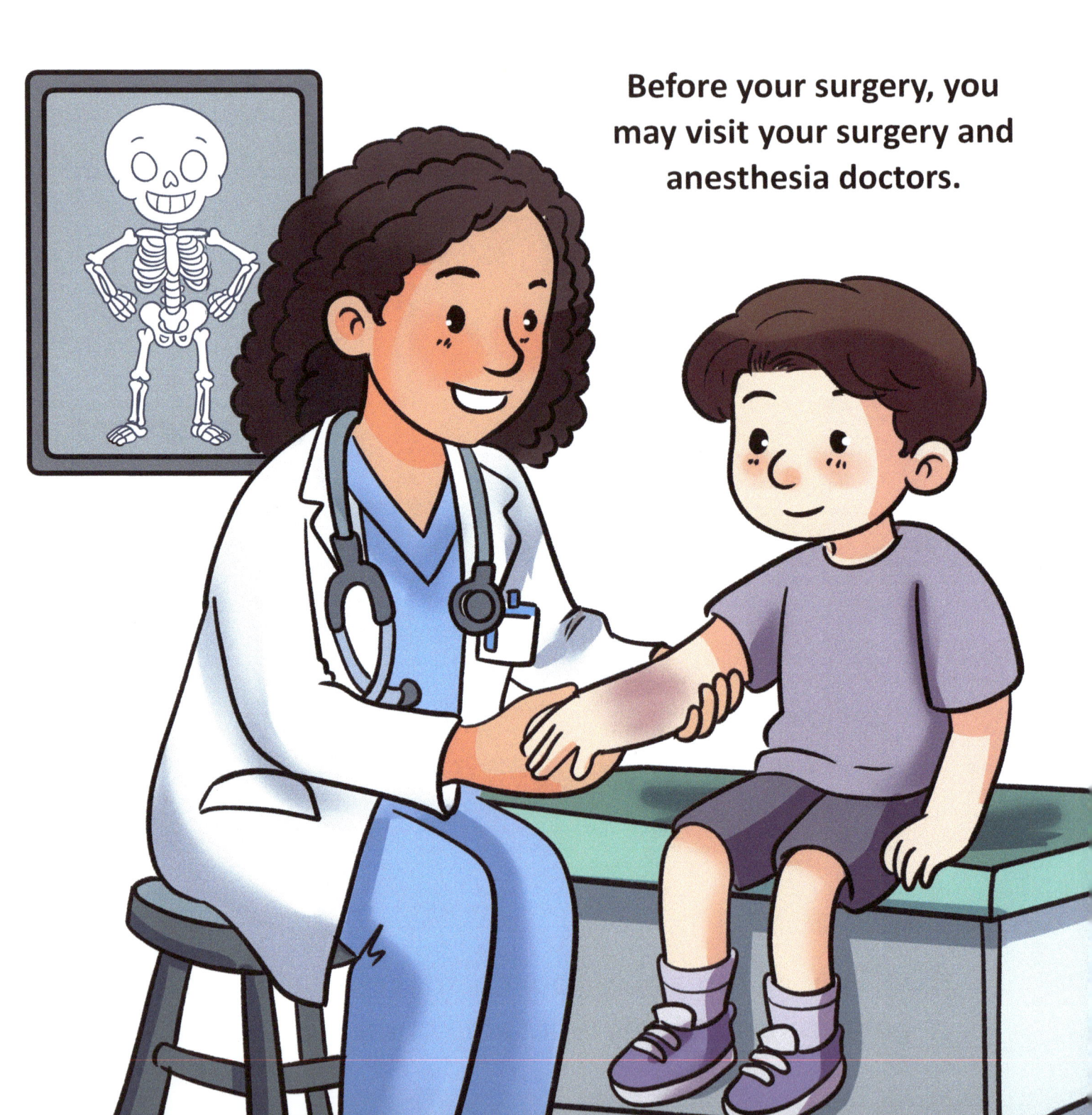

Before your surgery, you may visit your surgery and anesthesia doctors.

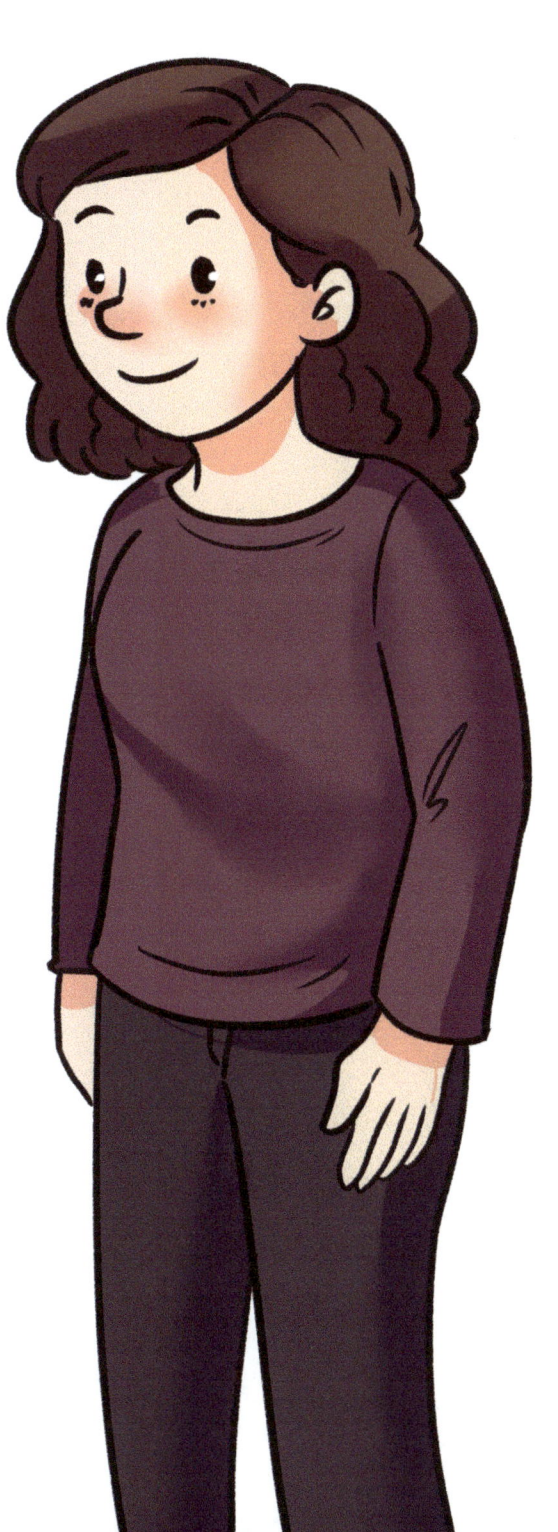

They'll help you learn how your bone will be fixed and what you can do to help it heal.

You'll also find out how to get ready for your anesthesia and surgery.

You can do this!

On surgery day, you won't eat breakfast.
That's how your body gets ready for the big day!

You can bring something special from home like your favorite toy, blanket, or book.

It's okay to feel a little nervous. Everyone does sometimes!

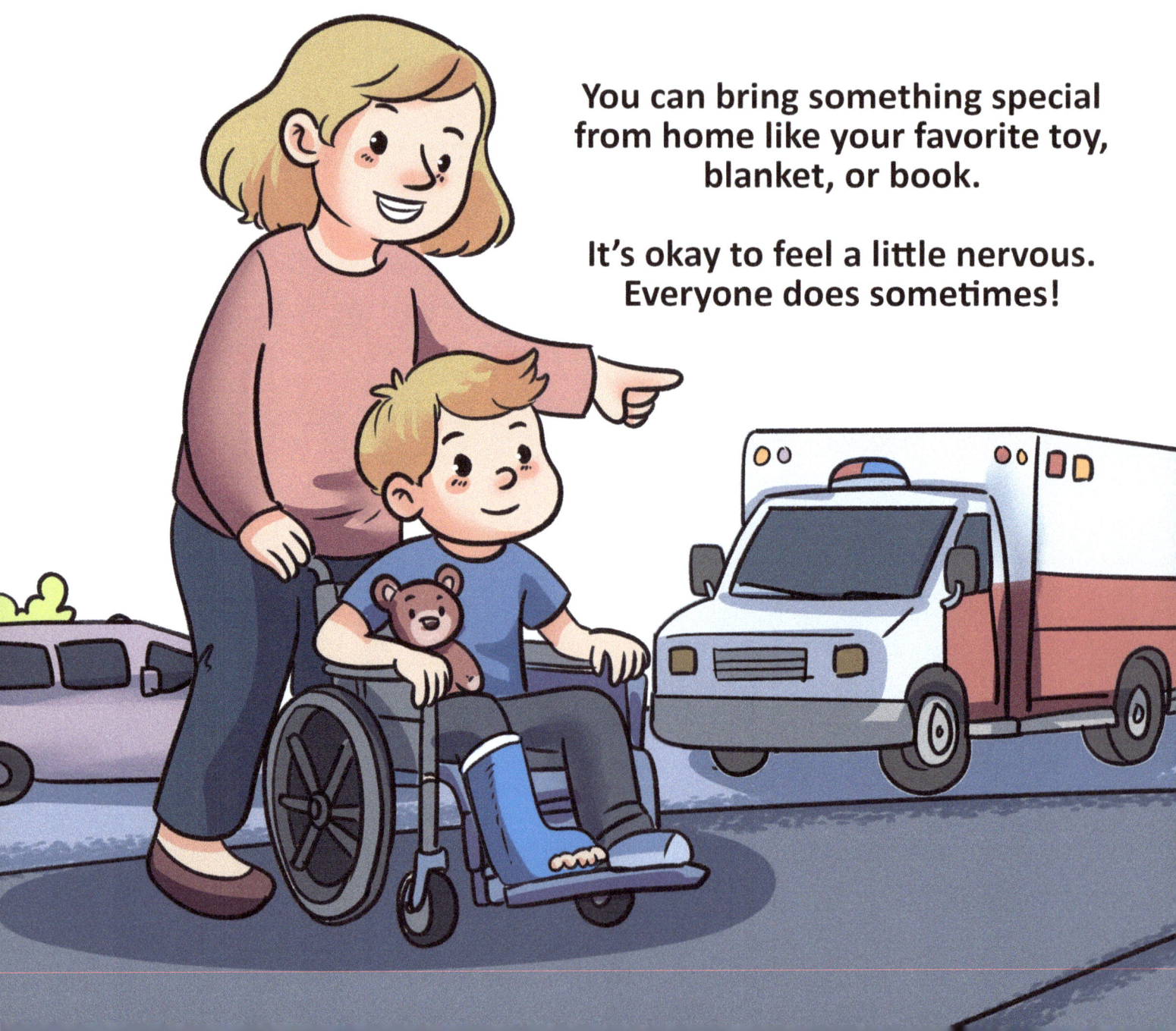

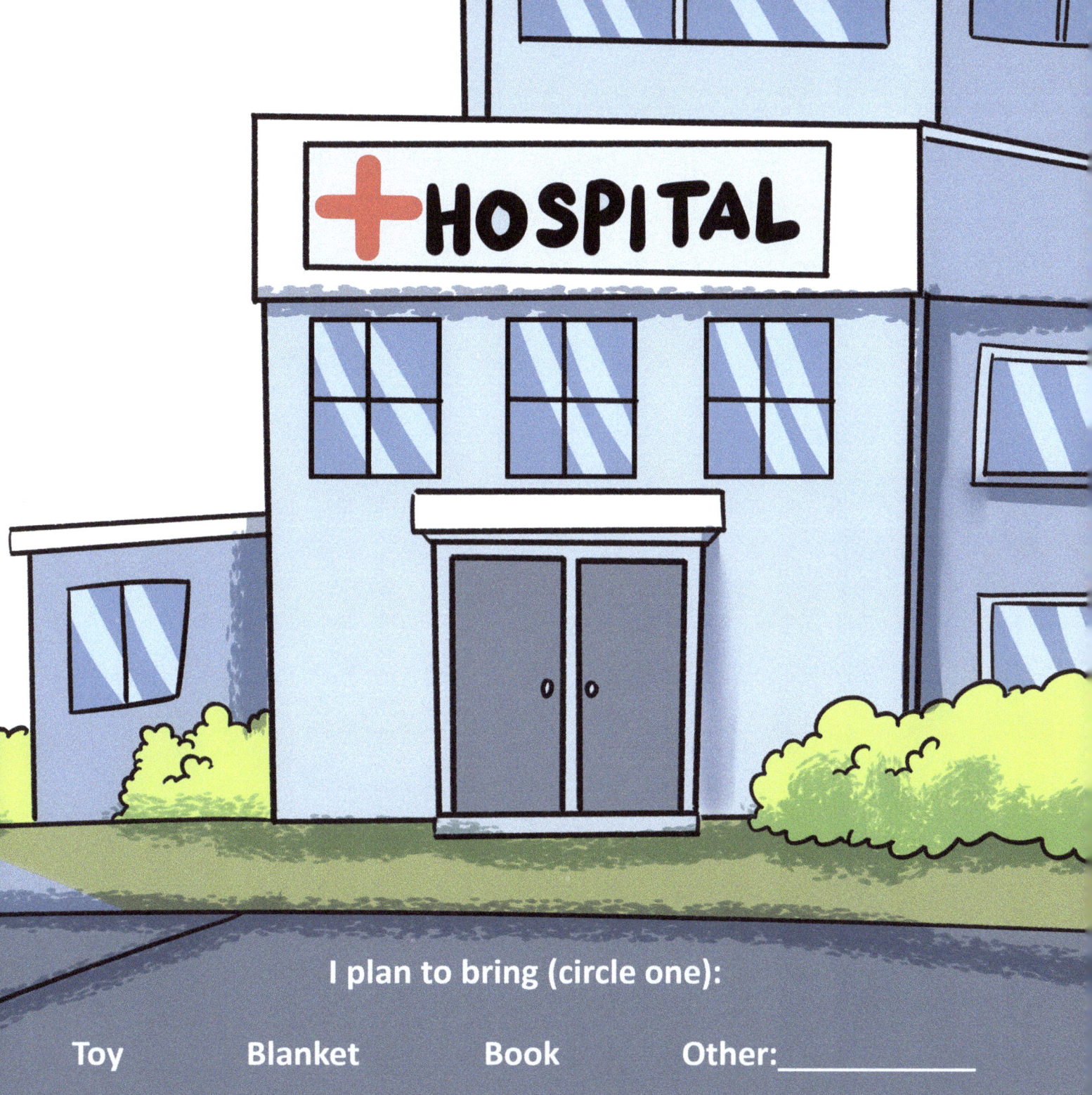

I plan to bring (circle one):

Toy			Blanket			Book			Other:_____

You'll check in and tell them your name and birthday.

They'll give you a special wristband so that everyone will know your name.

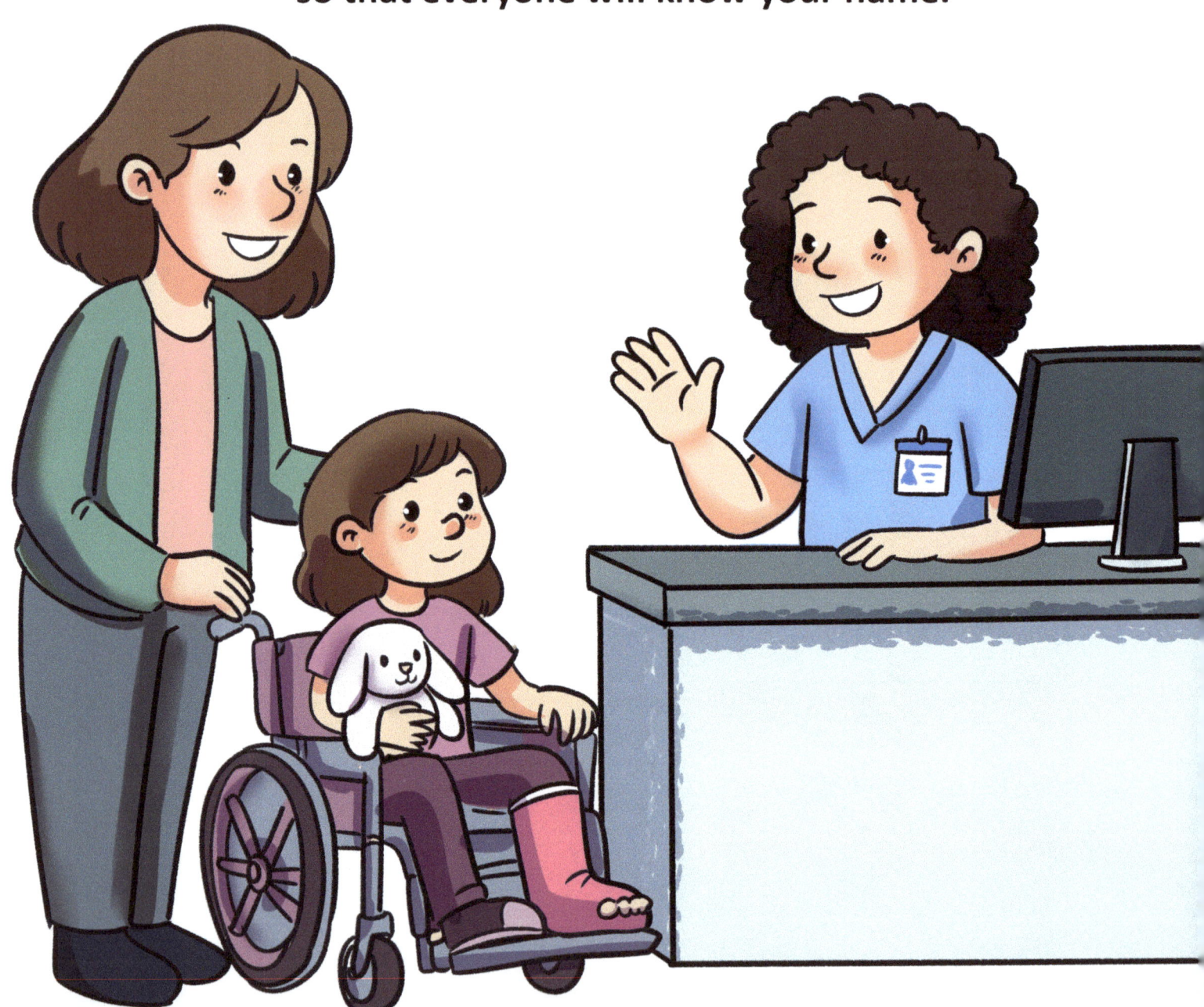

What color wristband will you get?
Circle the color of your wristband below.

Red Green Yellow Blue Pink Orange

Purple Black White

Other: _____

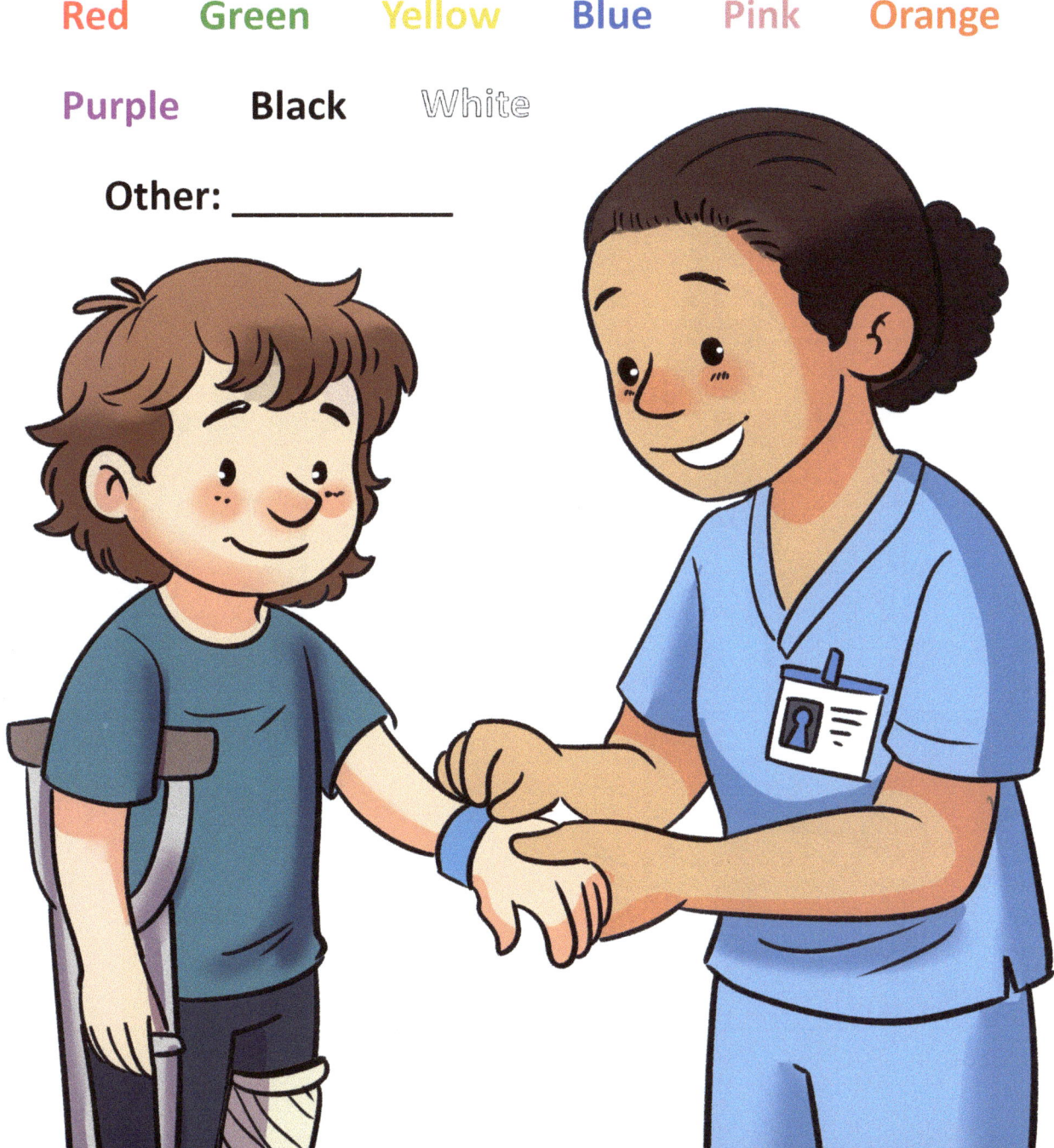

They will check your weight and height.

Do you know how much you weigh?
Do you know how tall you are?

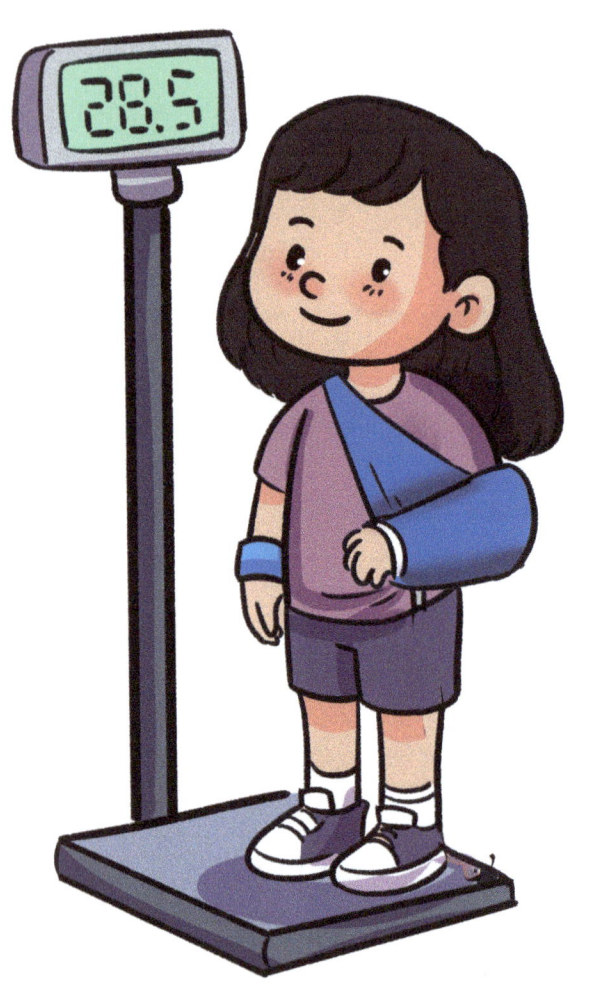
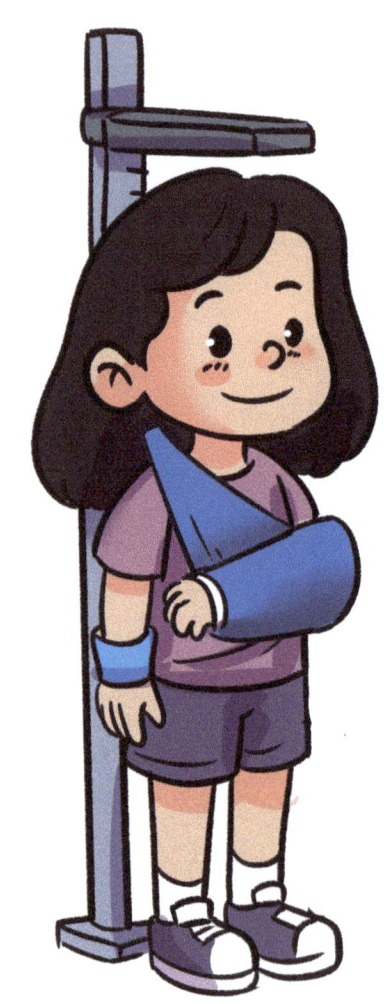

My weight is: _____   My height is: _____

You will change into a new outfit, put on a hat, a gown (it's like a backward superhero cape!), and some cozy socks.

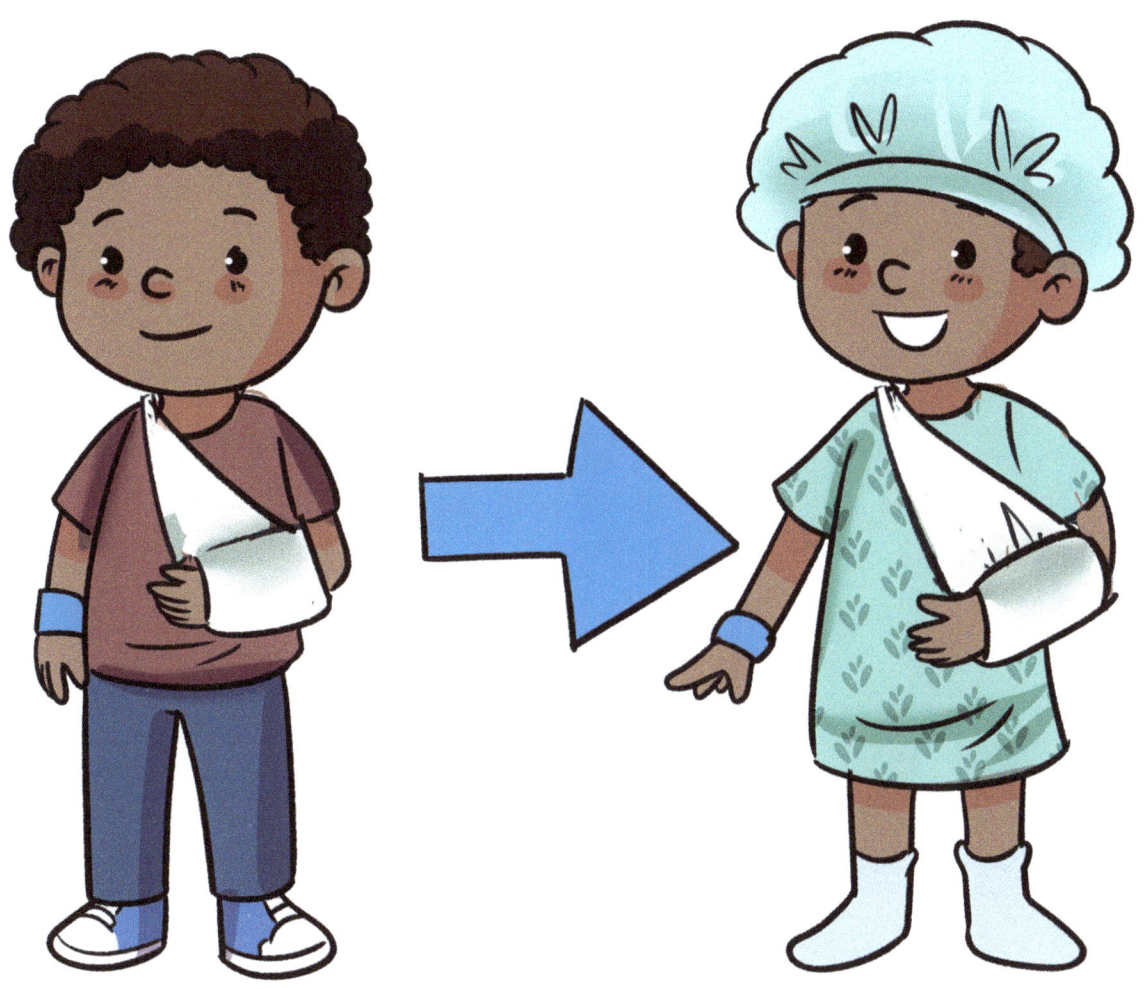

You've got this!

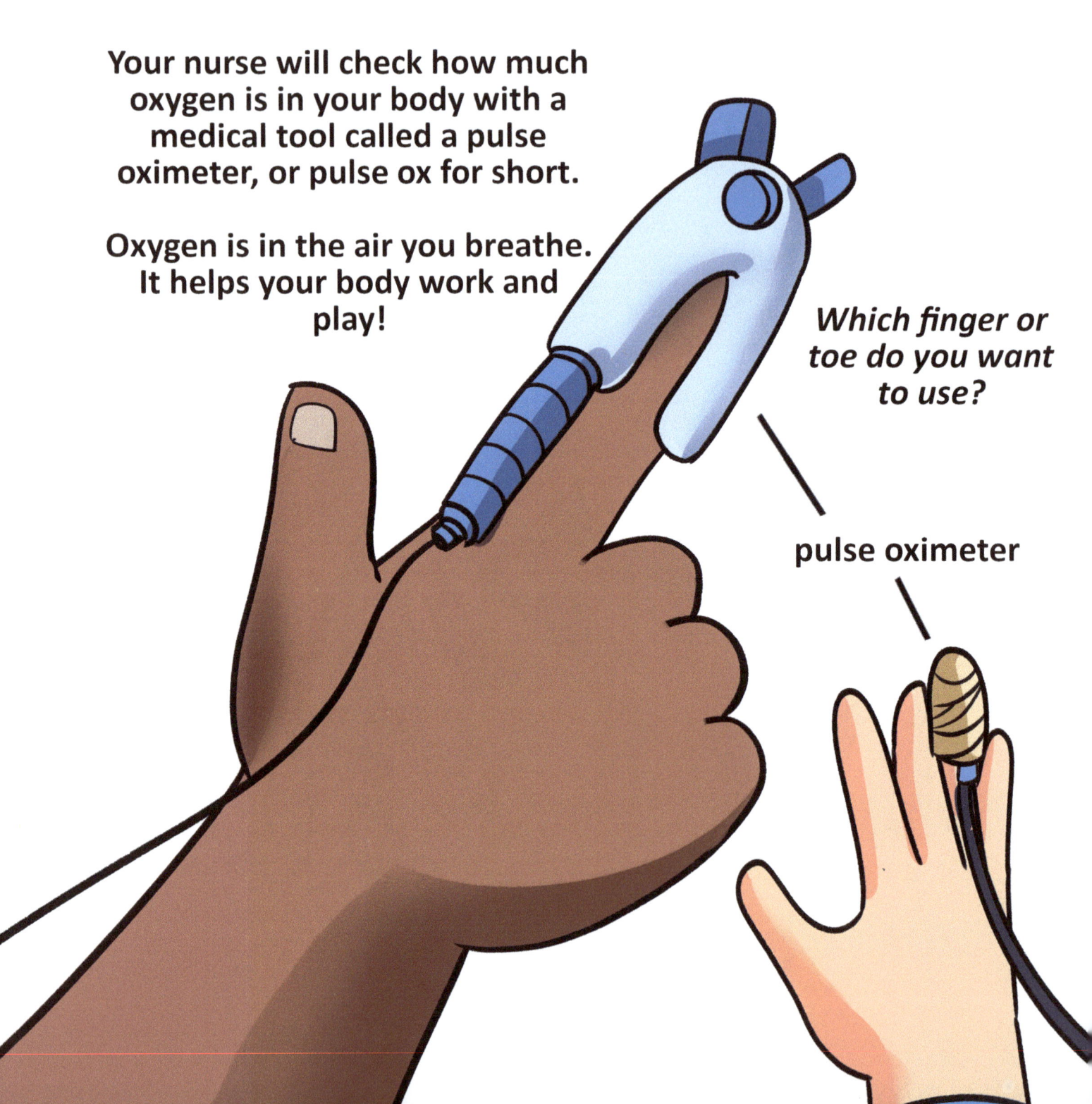

Your nurse will check how much oxygen is in your body with a medical tool called a pulse oximeter, or pulse ox for short.

Oxygen is in the air you breathe. It helps your body work and play!

Which finger or toe do you want to use?

pulse oximeter

You'll get a blood pressure cuff around your arm or leg.
It will give you a BIG hug!
Remember to stay still.

Are you ready?

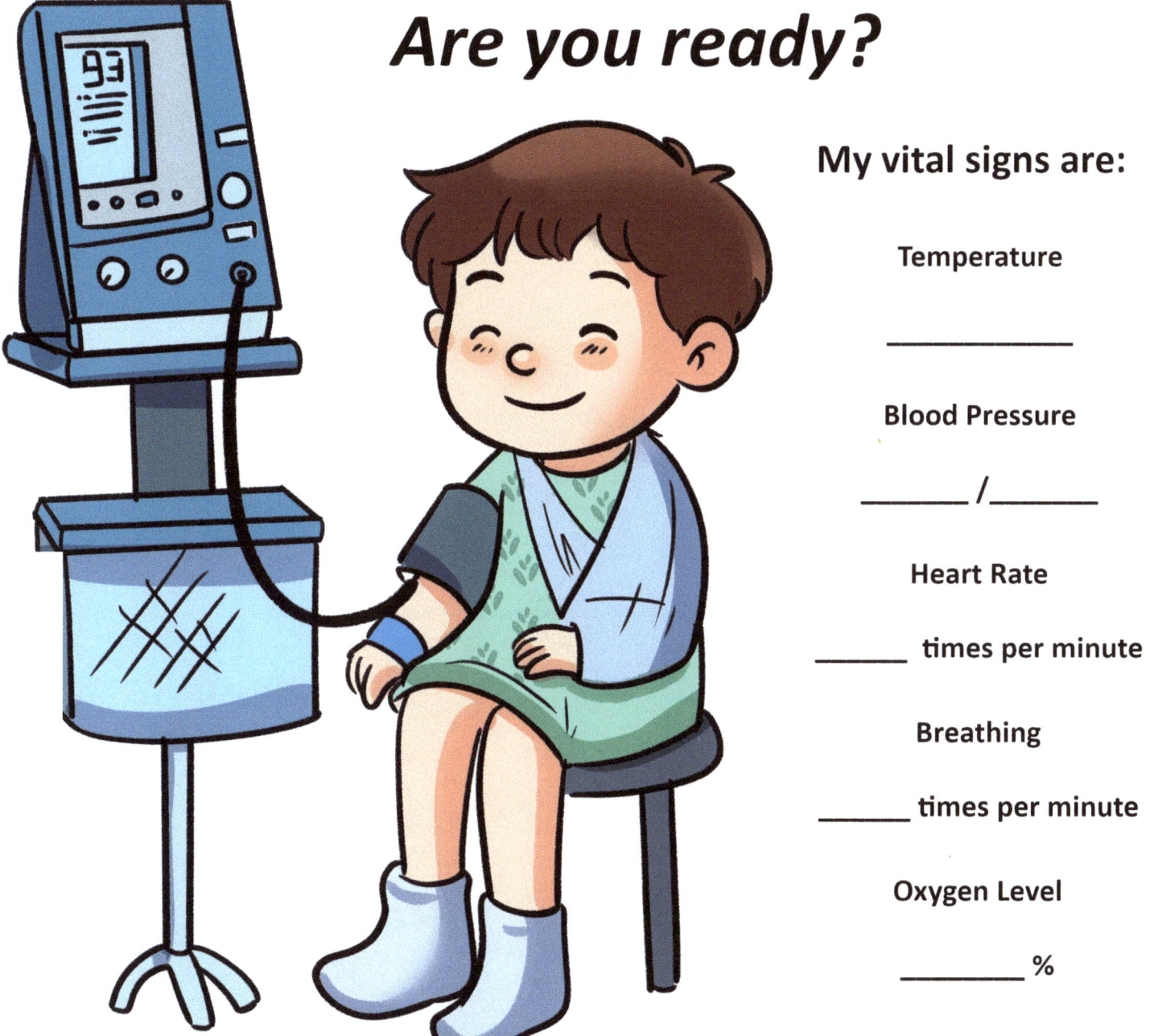

My vital signs are:

Temperature

_____

Blood Pressure

_____ / _____

Heart Rate

_____ times per minute

Breathing

_____ times per minute

Oxygen Level

_____ %

You and your grown-up will meet your doctors and nurses. They're friendly, kind, and here to help you feel better!

Also, they are happy to answer any questions you have. If you have any questions, please feel free to ask!

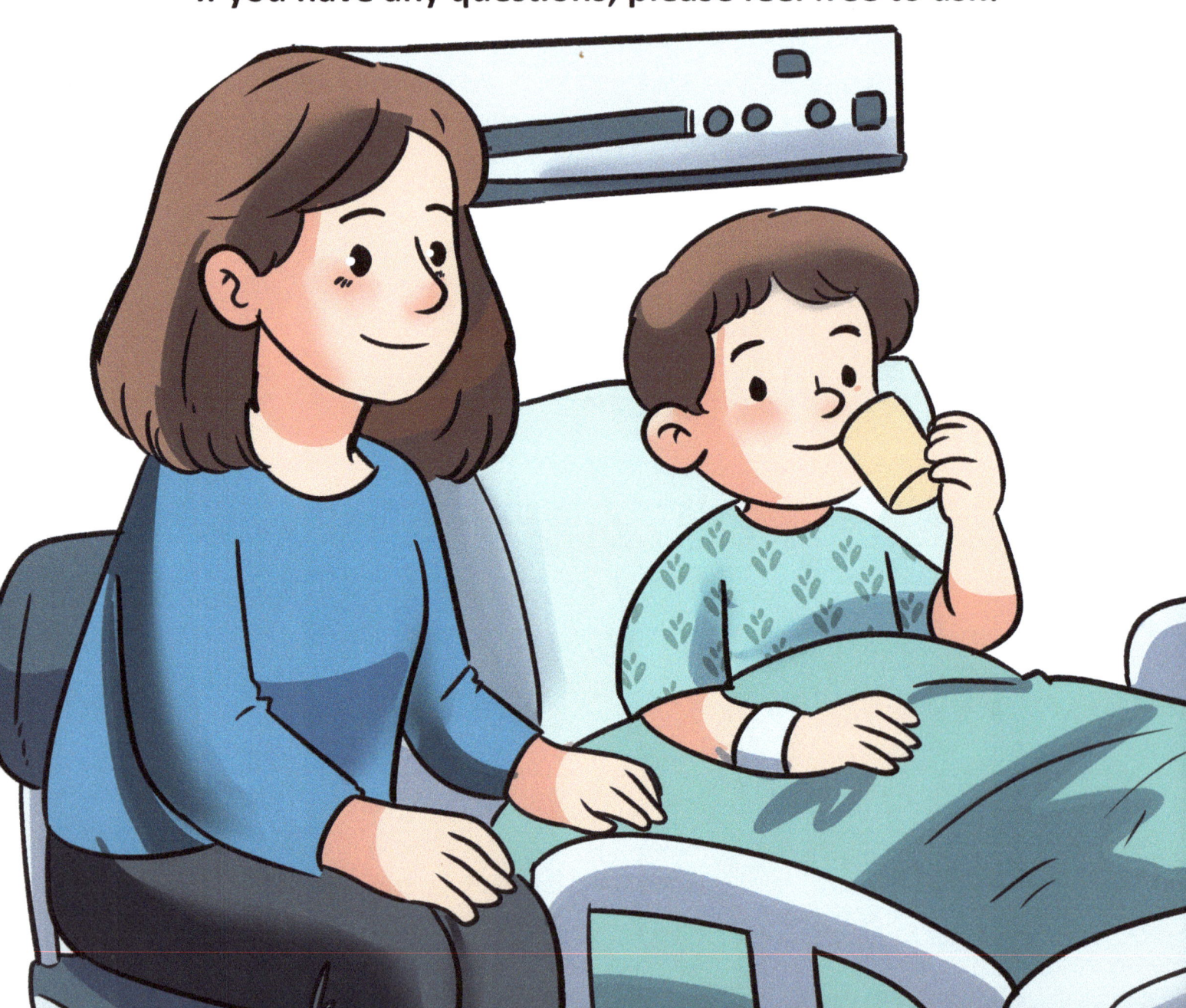

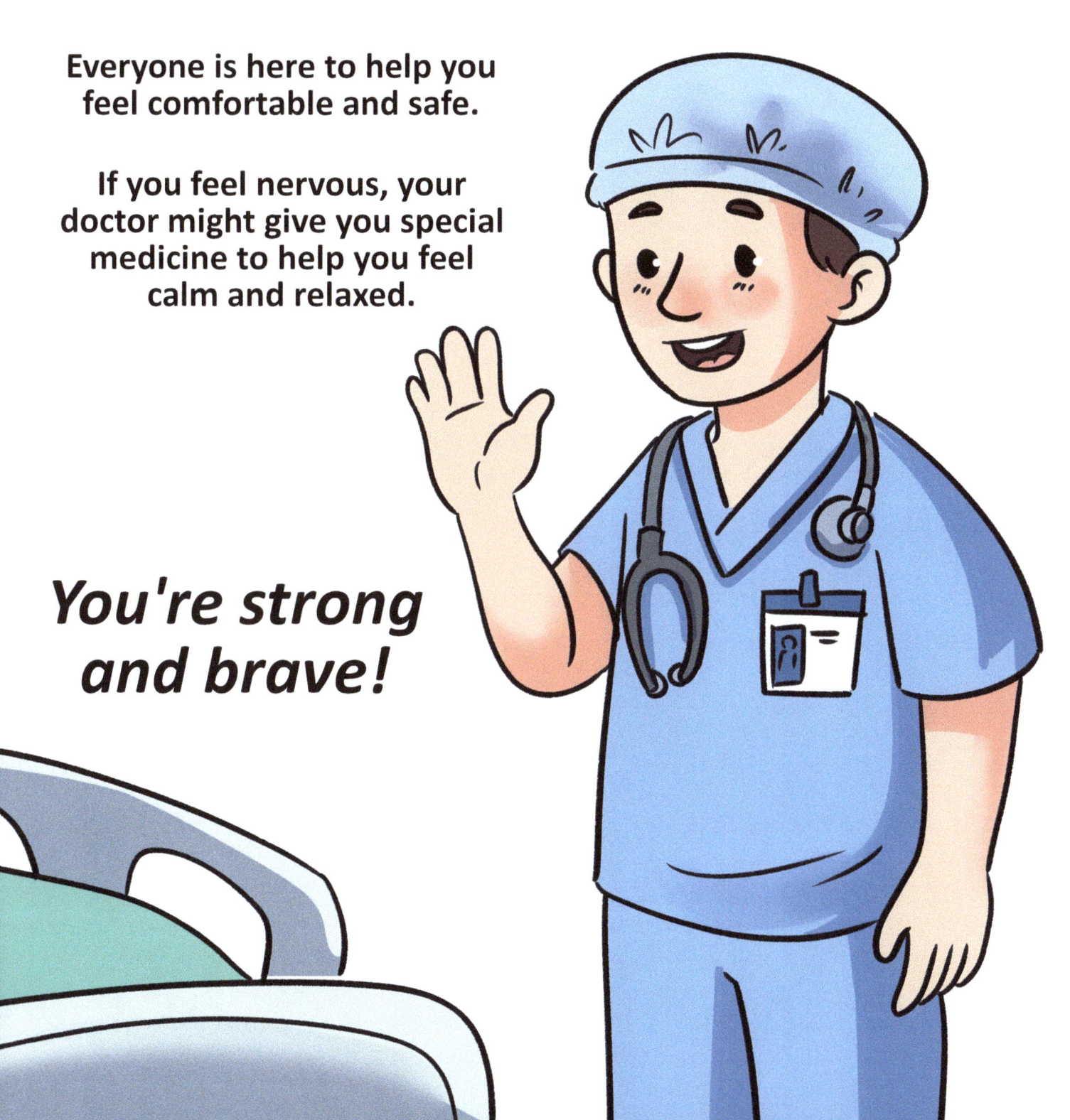

Everyone is here to help you feel comfortable and safe.

If you feel nervous, your doctor might give you special medicine to help you feel calm and relaxed.

You're strong and brave!

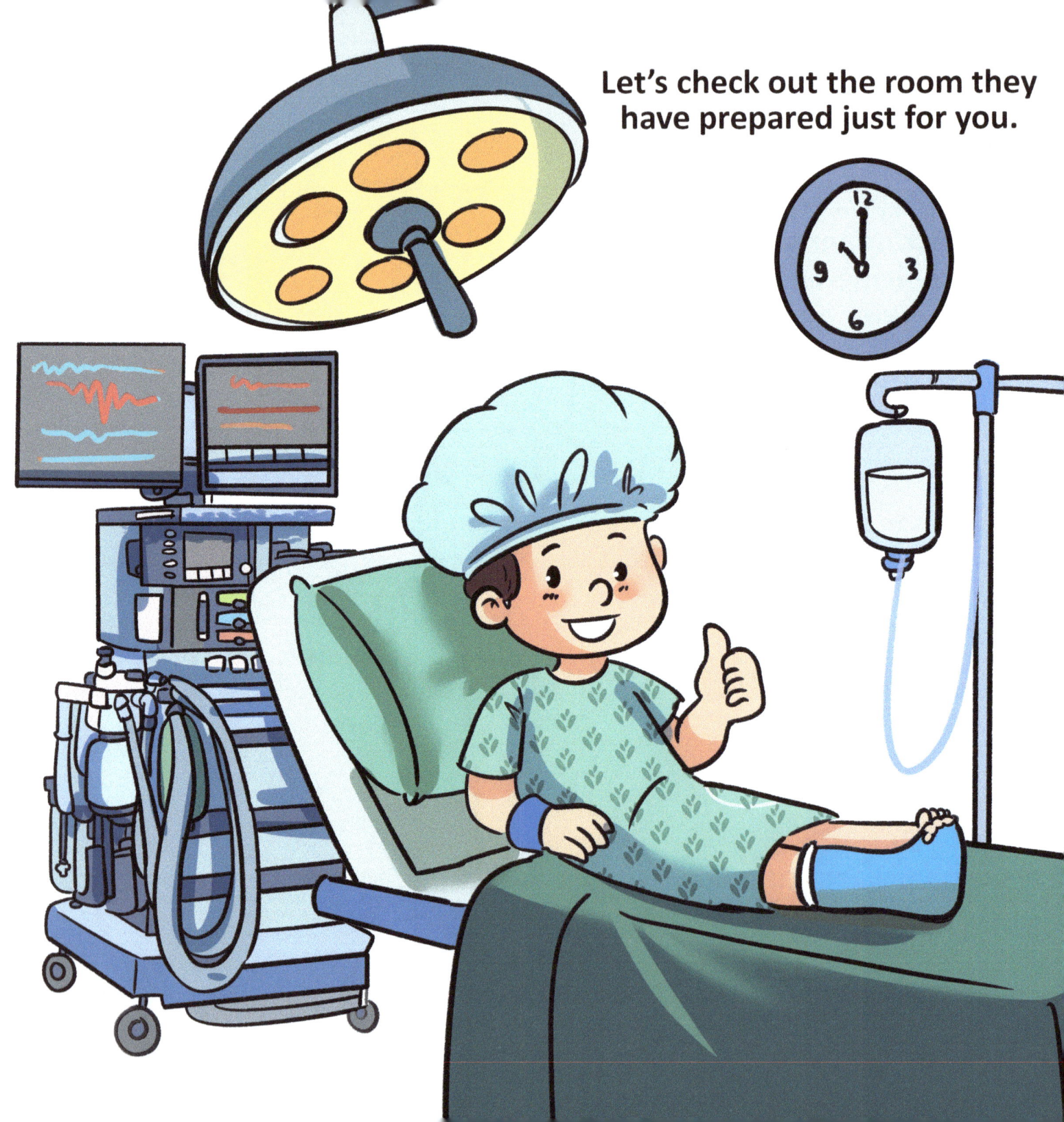

Can you find these things?

- [ ] A long table in the middle of the room just for you
- [ ] Friendly staff wearing masks
- [ ] Bright lights hanging from the ceiling
- [ ] An IV pole holding medicine or fluids
- [ ] A clock on the wall
- [ ] Boxes of gloves
- [ ] An anesthesia machine

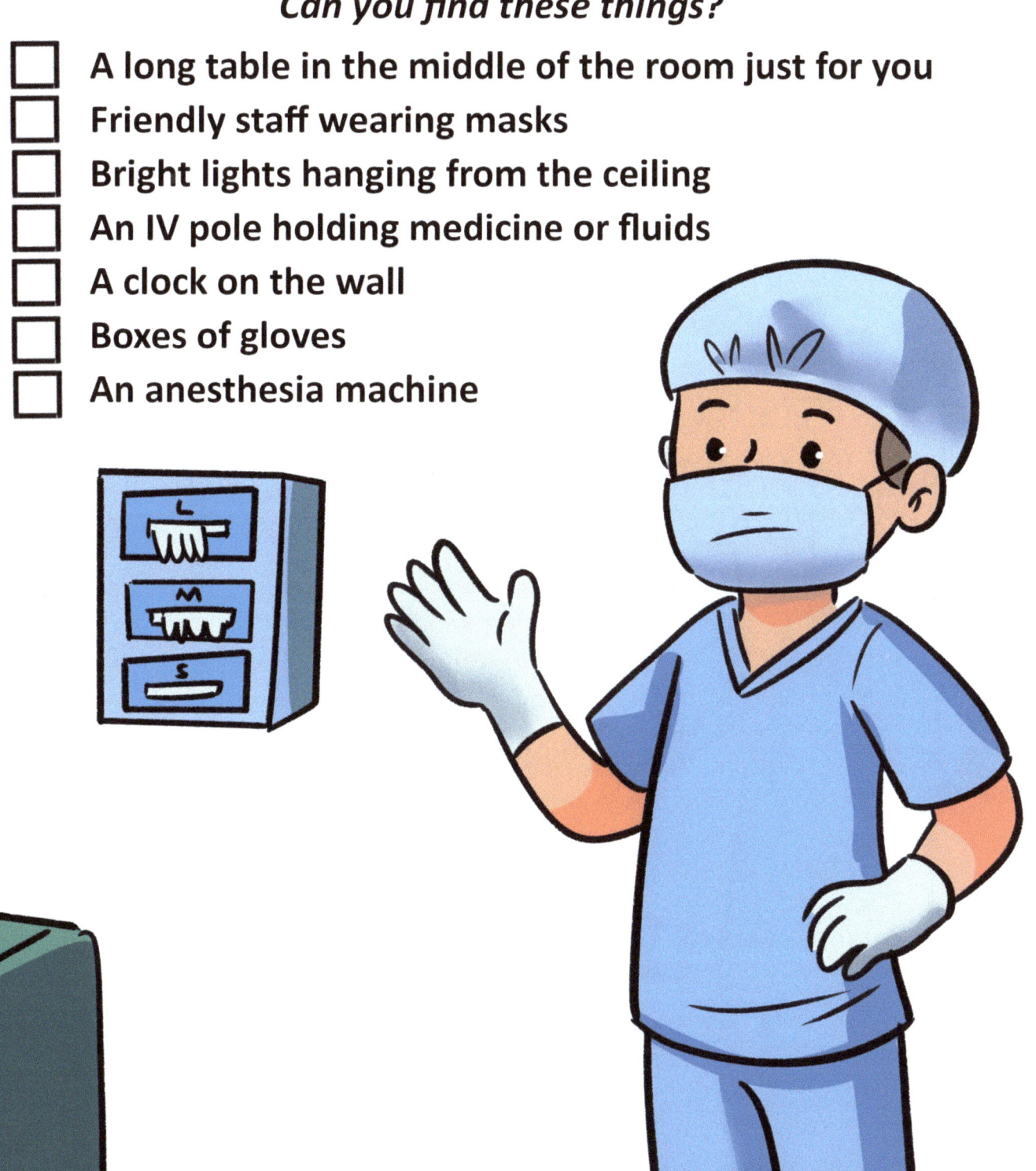

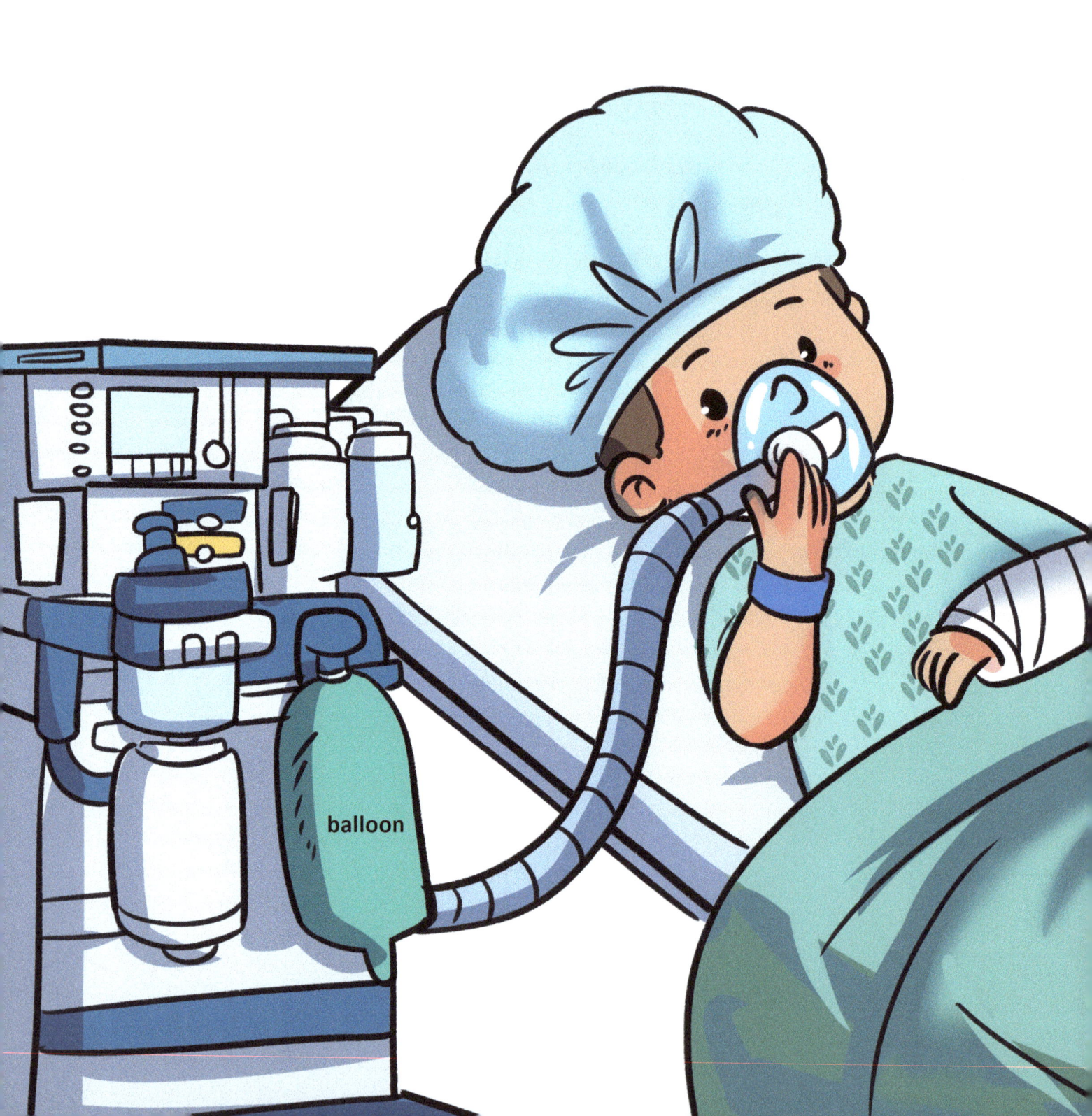

Your anesthesia doctor will give you a mask to breathe into.

Did you know they can make your mask smell sweet and delicious like bubble gum or your favorite fruit?

Draw or write what scent you'd like your mask to smell like:

_____

You can see your breathing by looking at the balloon attached to the anesthesia machine.

Cool, right?

<u>Challenge</u>: Can you count to ten before you fall asleep?
Let's try together!
1... 2... 3... 4... 5... 6... 7... 8... 9... 10...

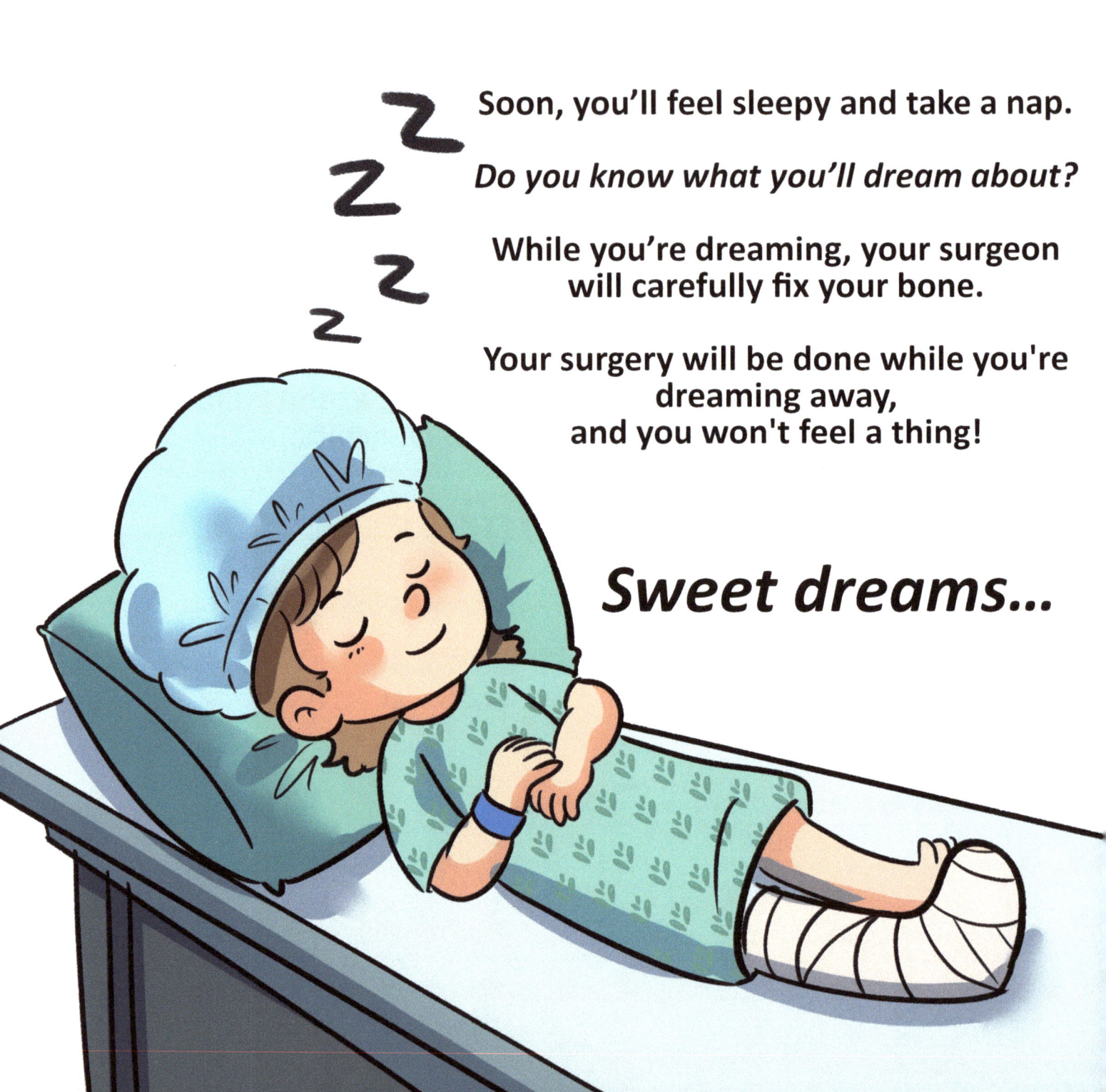

Your nurses and doctors will keep you safe and comfortable the whole time.

You're so brave!

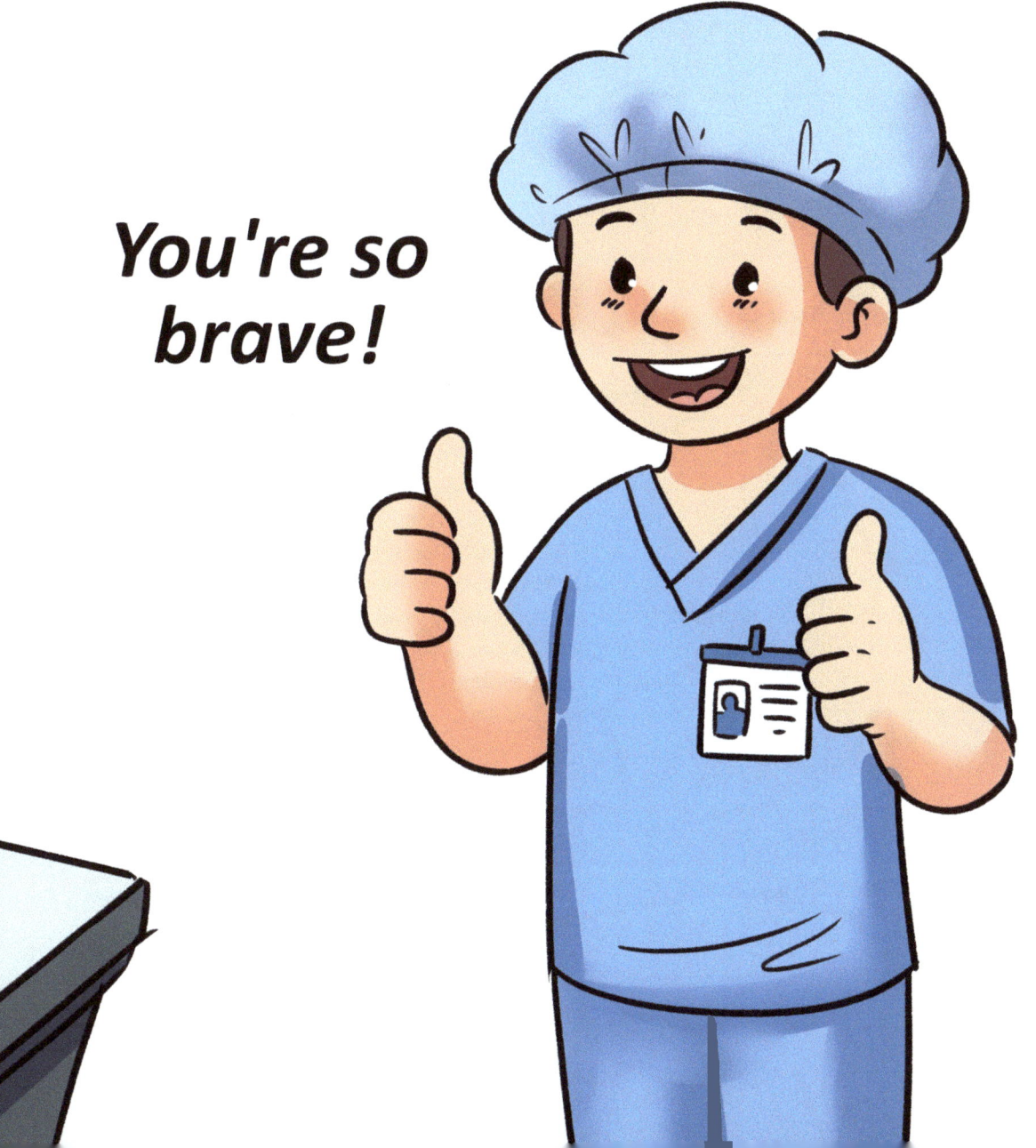

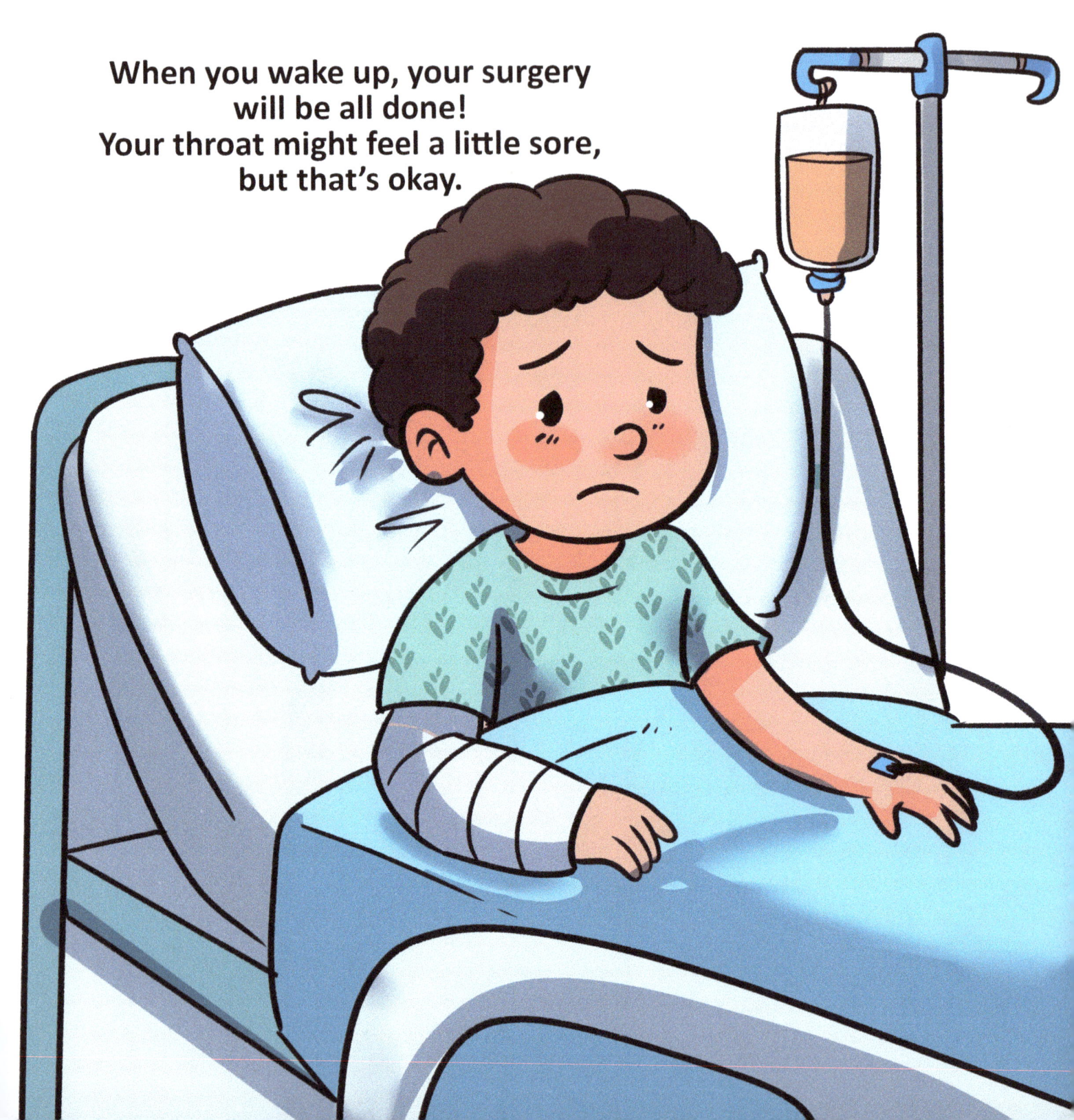

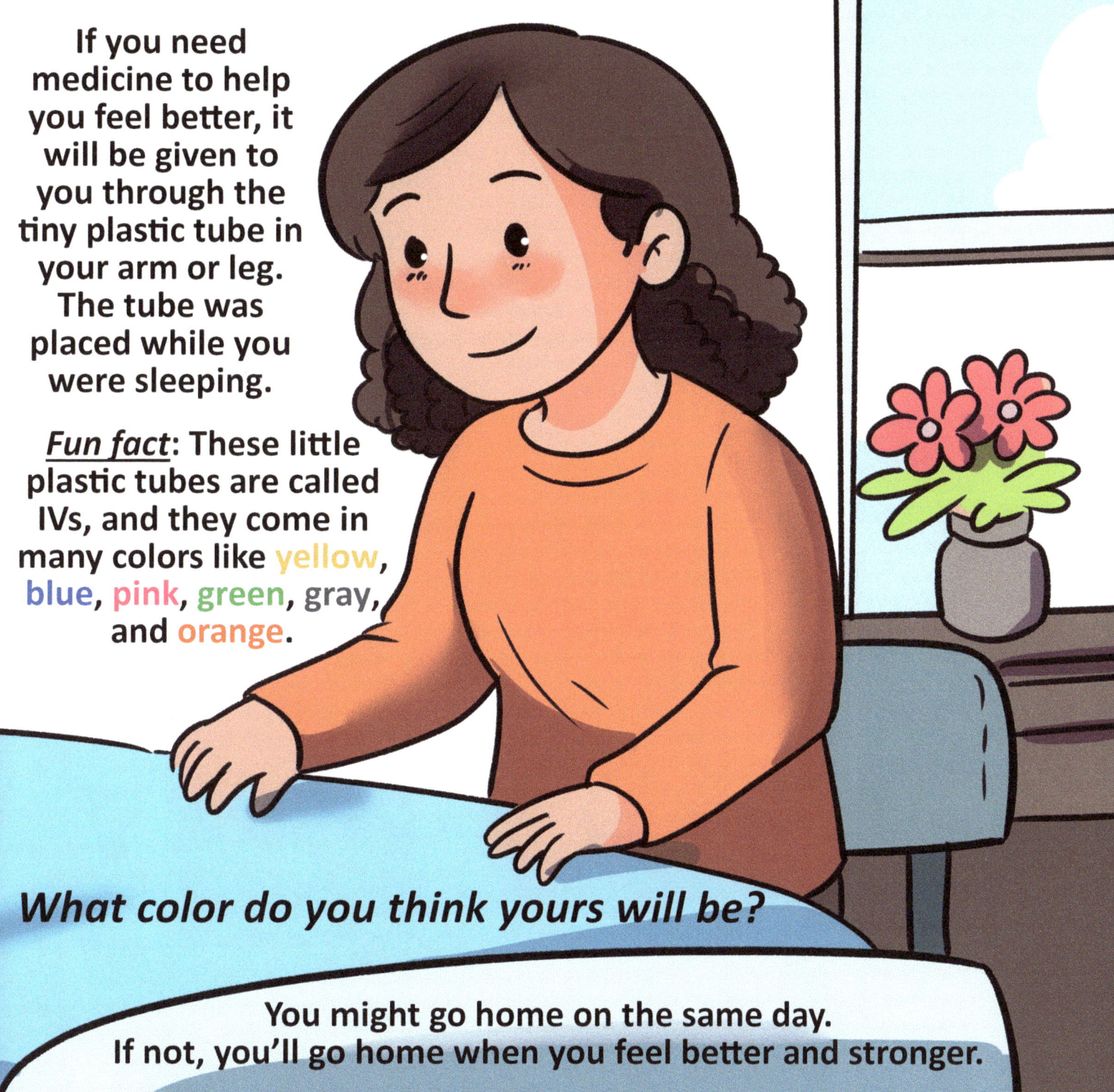

If you need medicine to help you feel better, it will be given to you through the tiny plastic tube in your arm or leg. The tube was placed while you were sleeping.

Fun fact: These little plastic tubes are called IVs, and they come in many colors like yellow, blue, pink, green, gray, and orange.

What color do you think yours will be?

You might go home on the same day.
If not, you'll go home when you feel better and stronger.

What are some things that will help you feel better and more comfortable after your surgery?
Place a checkmark (✓) next to your favorites!

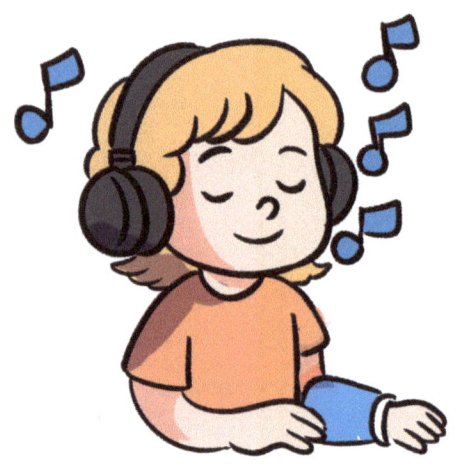

☐ listen to music

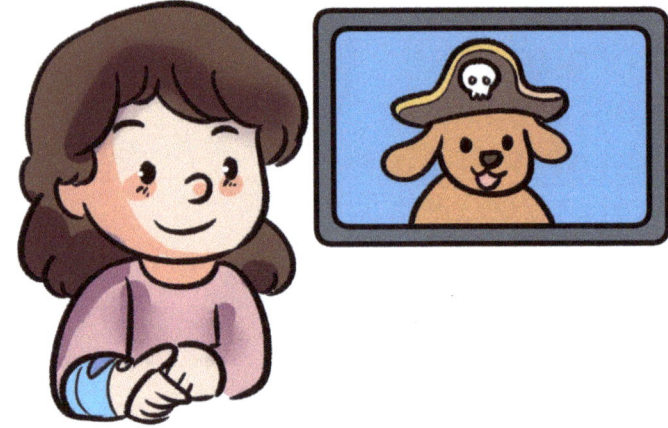

☐ watch your favorite show

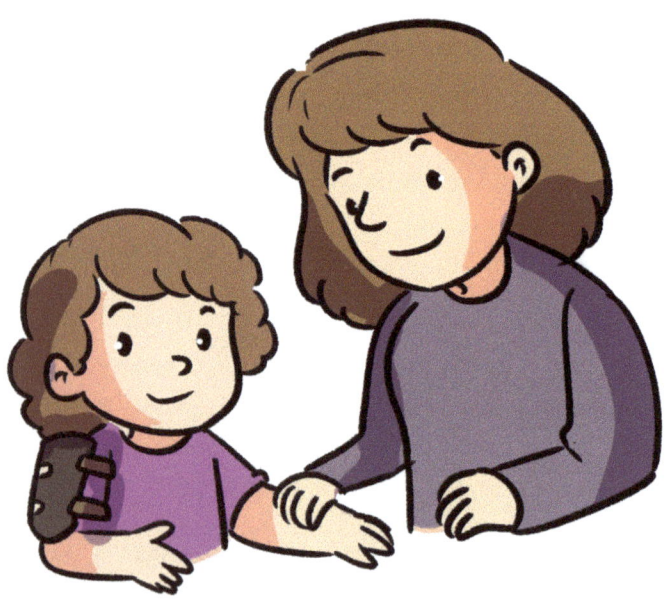

☐ get a gentle massage

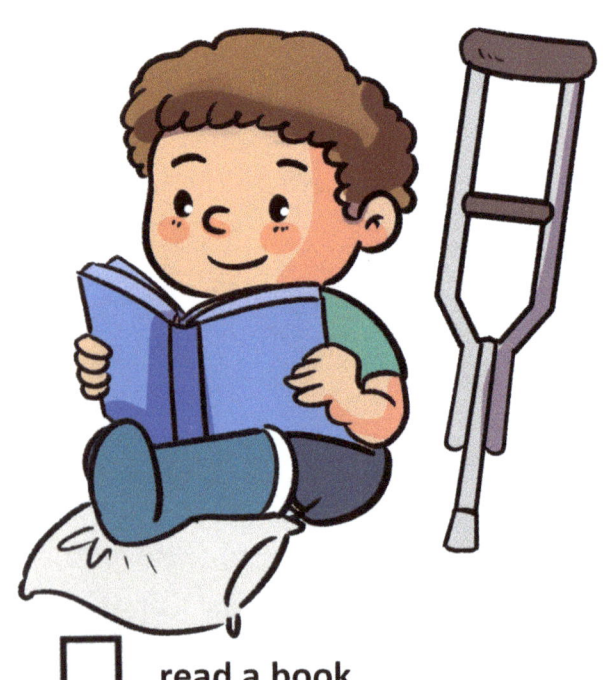

☐ read a book

What other creative ideas do you have to help you relax?

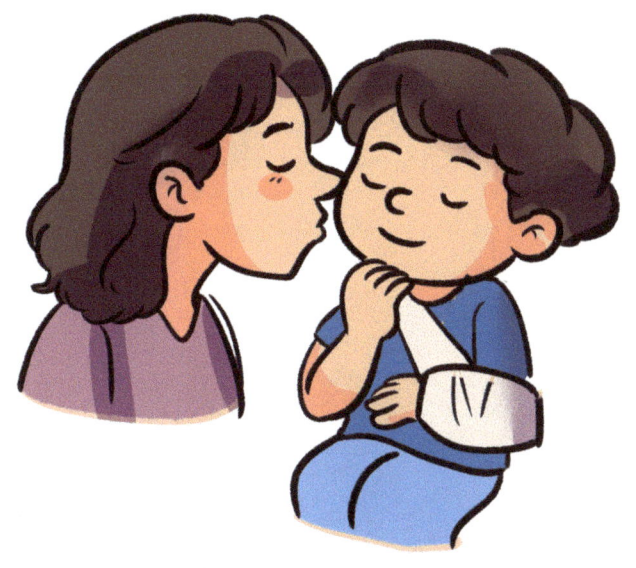

☐ get a sweet kiss

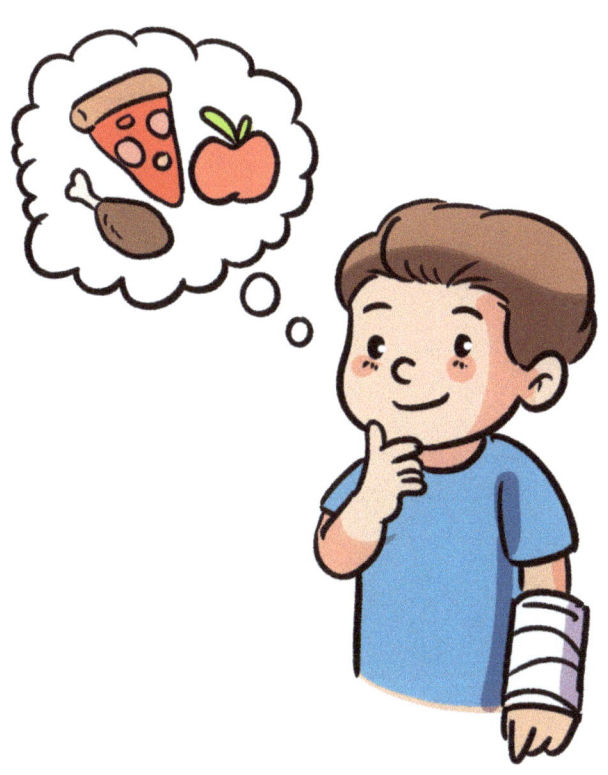

☐ think about what food you would like to eat when you feel better

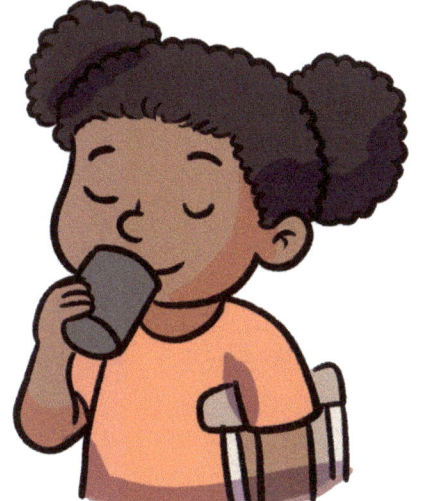

☐ take some medicine

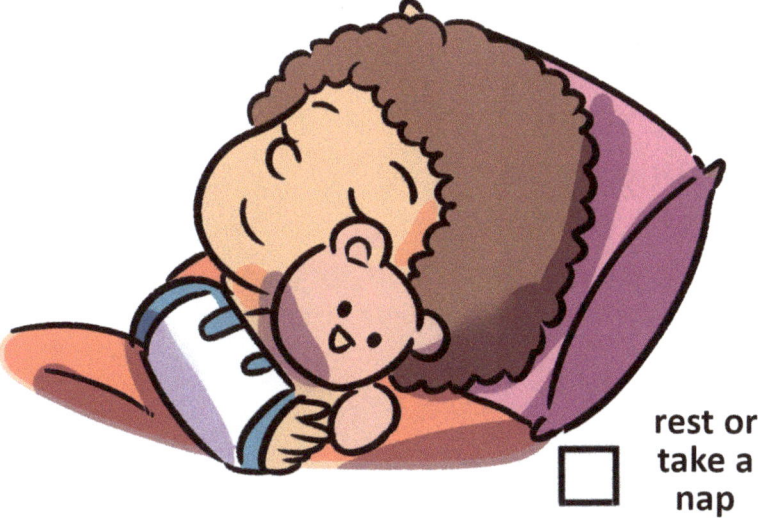

☐ rest or take a nap

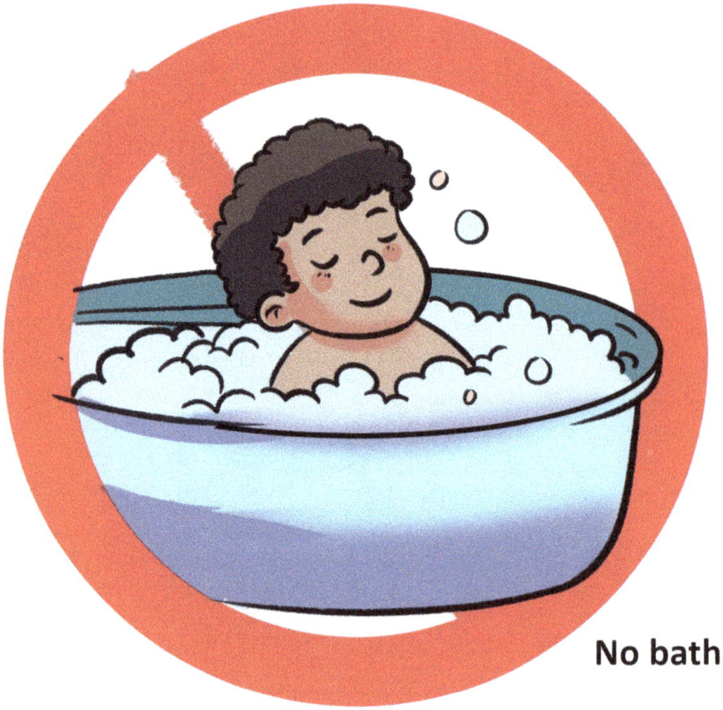

No bathing

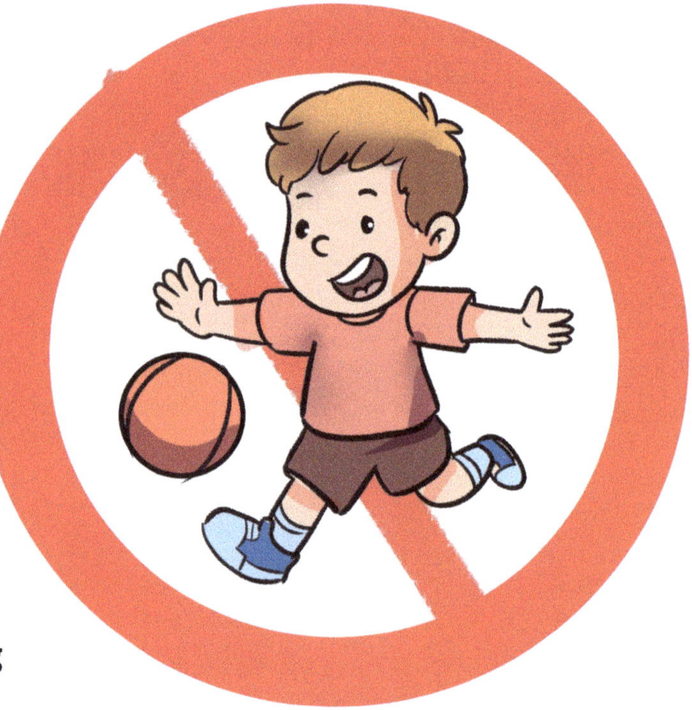

No contact sports (where players can bump into each other)

After your surgery, there might be some things you can't do for a little while until your body is ready.

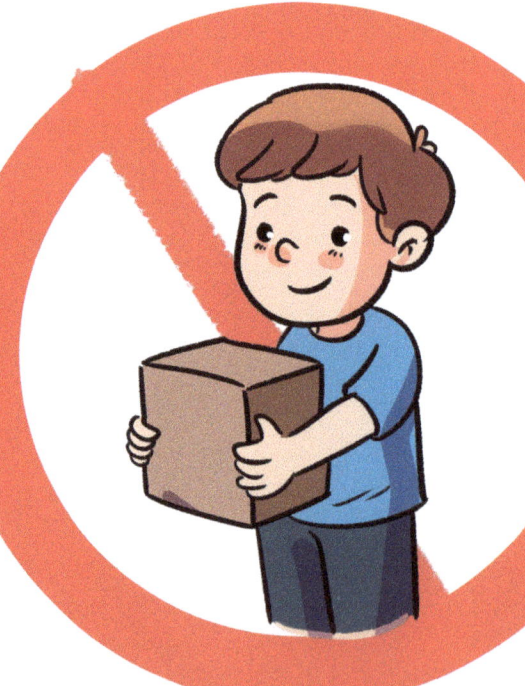

No heavy lifting

Your grown-up will help you keep your bandage clean and dry and remind you about the things you shouldn't do while you're healing.

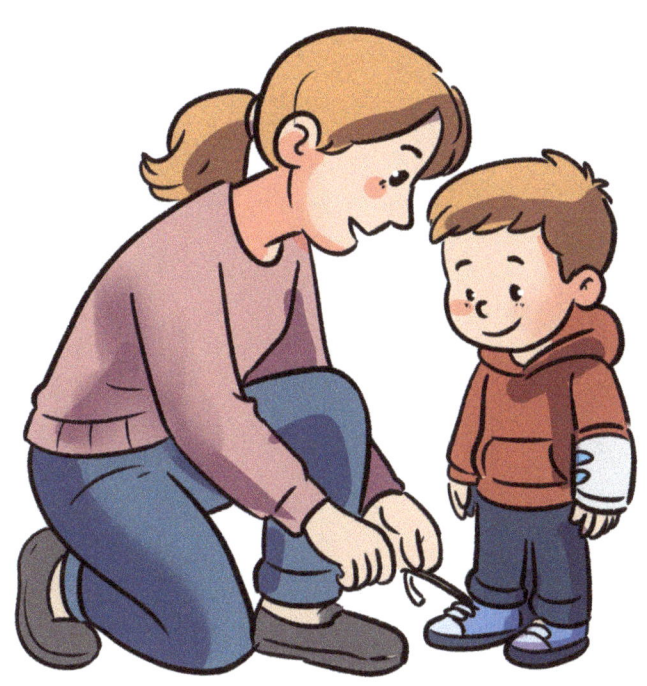

Don't worry!
Your doctor will tell your parent or guardian when it's safe to get back to your favorite activities.

Soon, you'll visit your doctor again to make sure your bone is healing well.

Your doctor will share ways to help you feel better, get strong, and stay healthy.

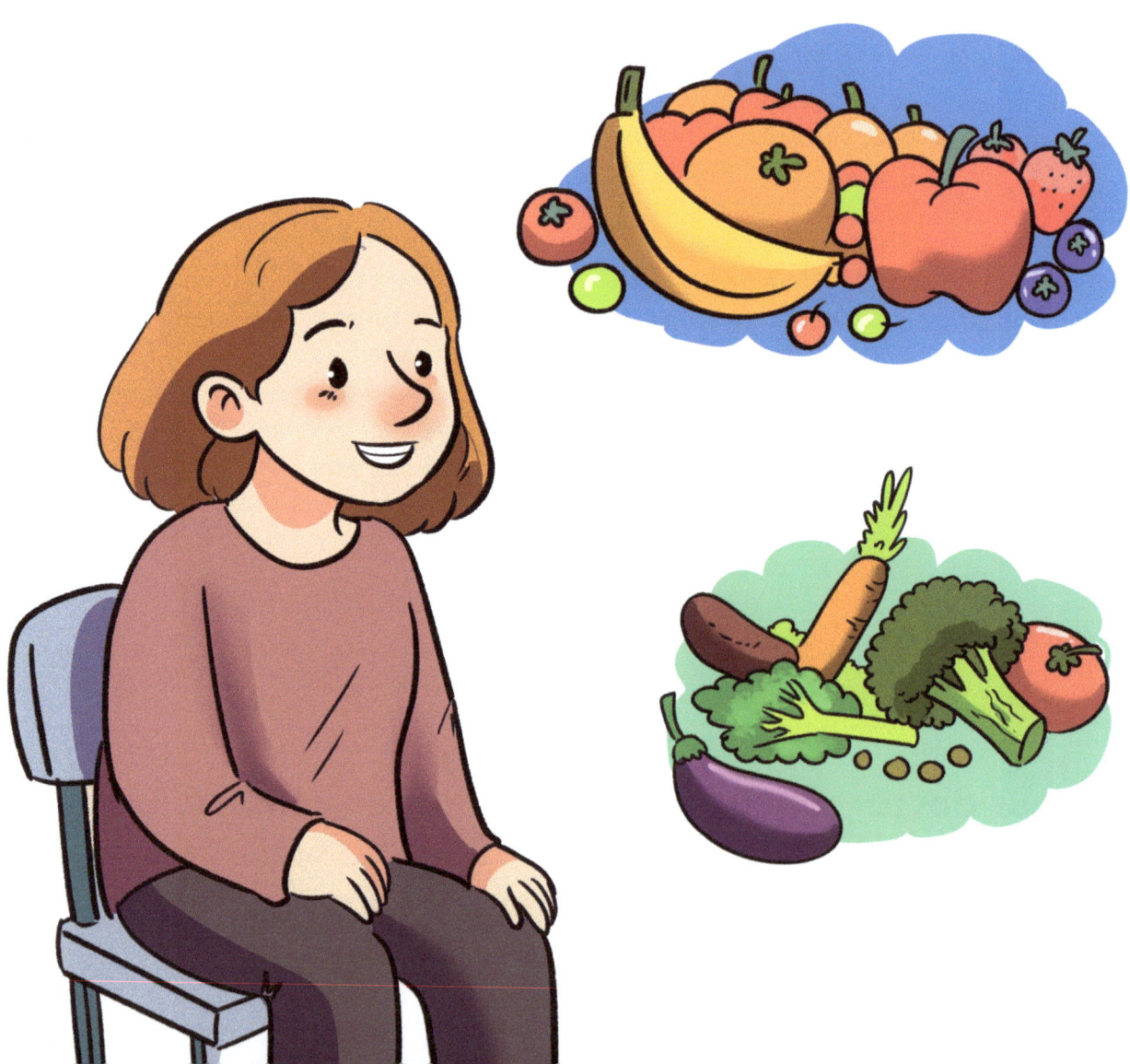

If you have any questions, your doctor is happy to help.

Write your questions below.

_____

_____

_____

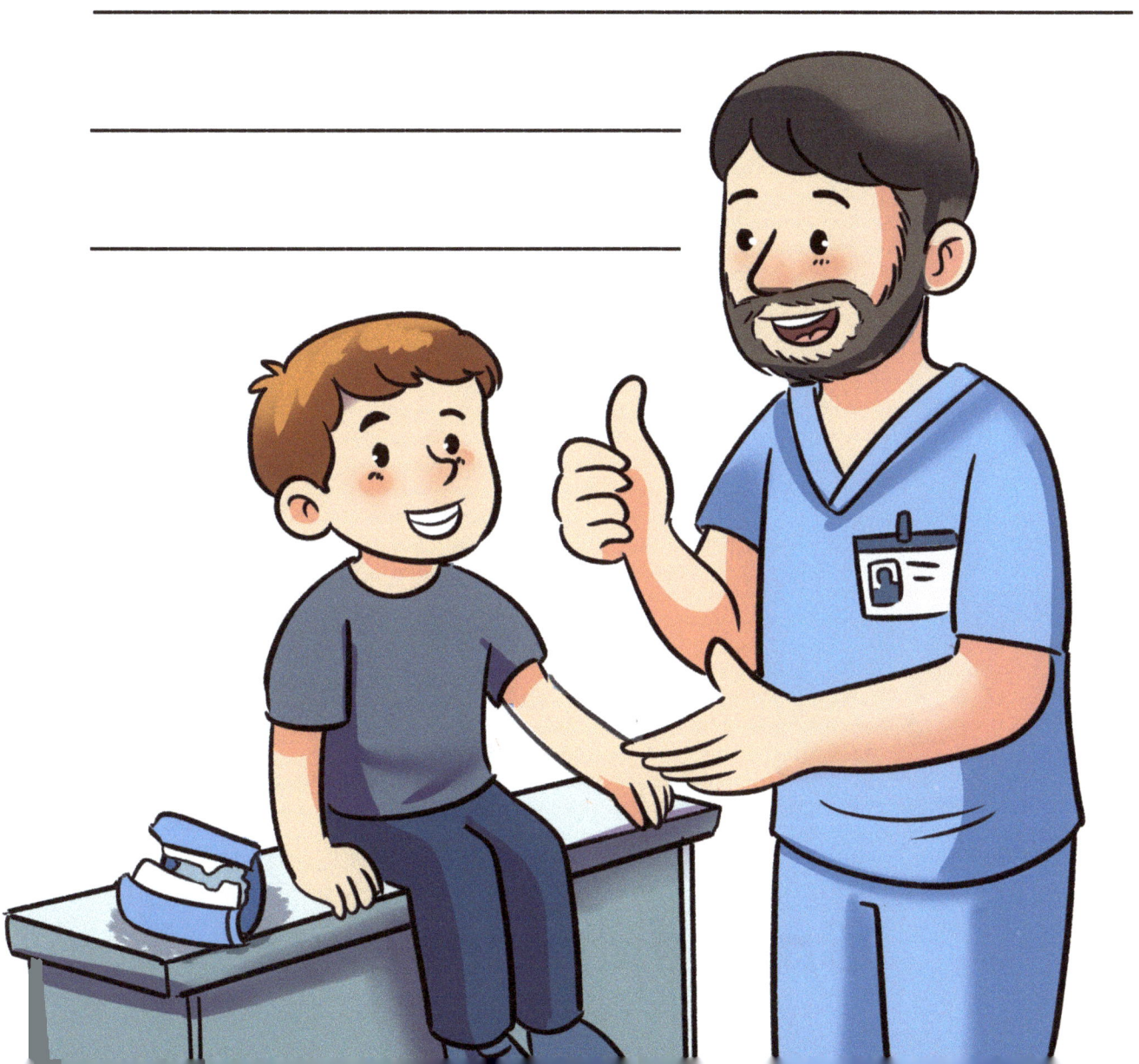

What will you do after your bone surgery?

A party? A celebration?

What's your favorite way to celebrate?

Draw or write your party plan below.

Speedy recovery!

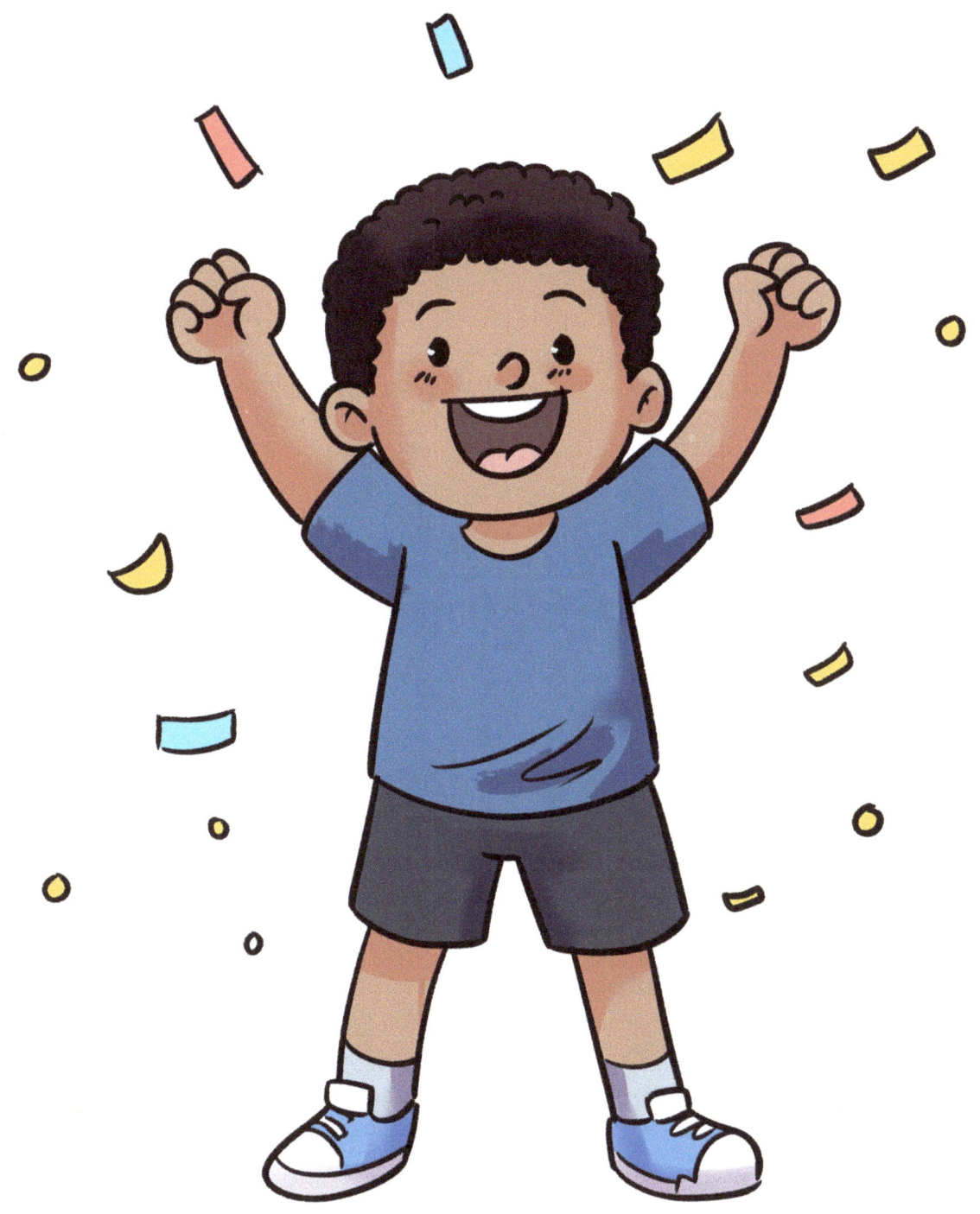

Notes for Parent/Guardian

- Placement of the intravenous (IV) catheter in this young age group is typically done *after* your child is asleep in the operating room.

- After the surgery, it is common for children to feel confused, disoriented, or irritable, and they may cry, sob, kick, scream, or thrash around. It normally takes about one hour for the anesthesia to wear off.

- Post-surgery instructions/restrictions:
Your child's doctor should give you specific instructions on (1) what your child can and cannot do during the recovery period, (2) the duration of the post-surgical restrictions, and (3) any post-surgical follow-ups. Additionally, (4) they should instruct what to watch out for and when it is necessary for you to bring your child back to the hospital in case of an emergency. If they forget, please kindly remind them and obtain these instructions/restrictions before leaving the hospital.

Disclaimer

Please note that the illustrations are not drawn to scale.

This book is written for informational, educational, and personal growth purposes and should not be used as a substitute for medical advice.

Please consult your child's doctor if they need medical attention and to ensure the information in this book pertains to your child's medical condition and needs. I cannot guarantee what your child experiences is exactly what is being discussed in this book.

The author and the publisher are not responsible, either directly or indirectly, for any damages, monetary losses, or reparations due to information in this book. By reading this book, the readers agree not to hold the author and the publisher responsible for any losses as a result of any errors, inaccuracies, or omissions in this book.

Please keep in mind that your child's experience depends on the location, the facility, their medical condition, and the healthcare team. Please use this book in conjunction with your child's doctor's advice. Thank you.

Did this picture book help your child in some way?
If so, I would love to hear about it!

www.amazon.com/gp/product-review/B0G1LVQ71N

For other book titles, please visit:

www.fzwbooks.com

Connect with the author

email: books@fzwbooks.com
facebook/instagram: @FZWbooks

Books by the author

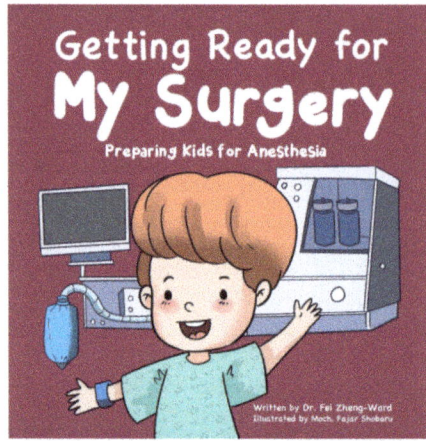
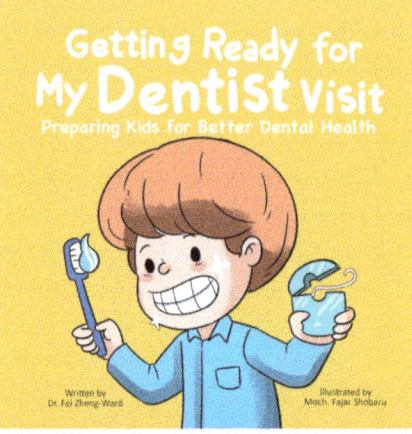
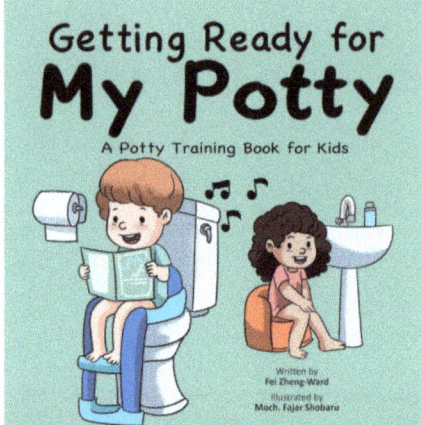
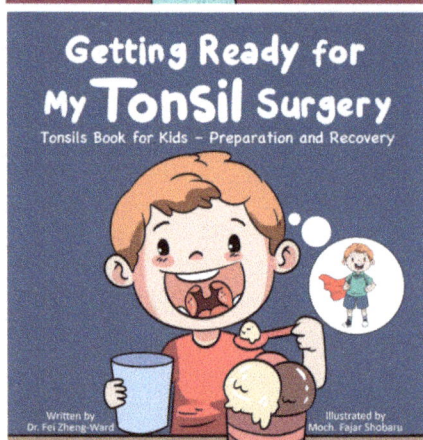
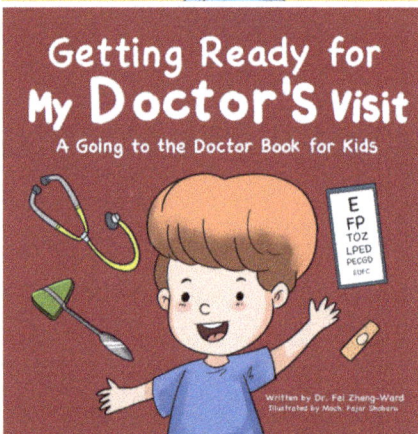
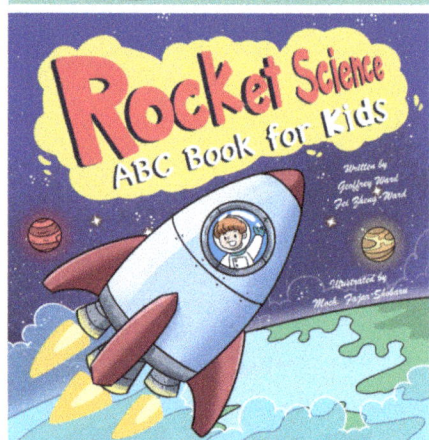
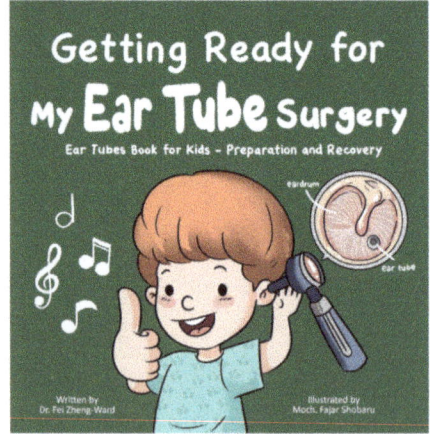
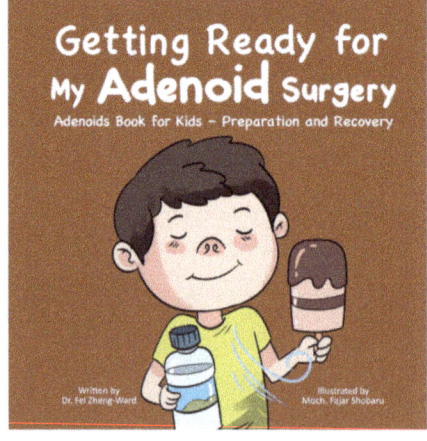
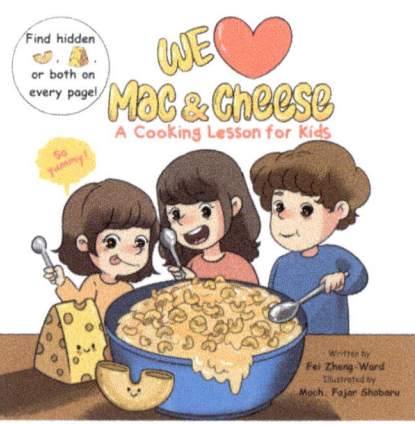

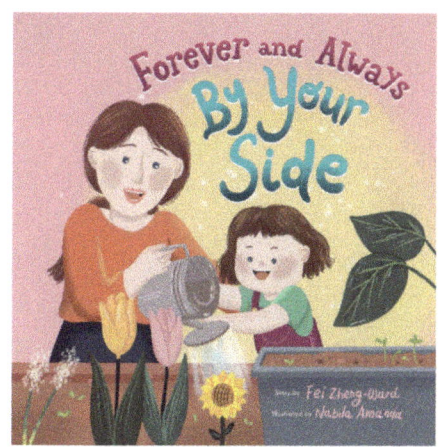
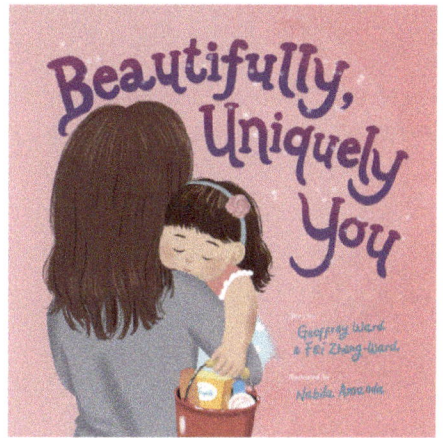
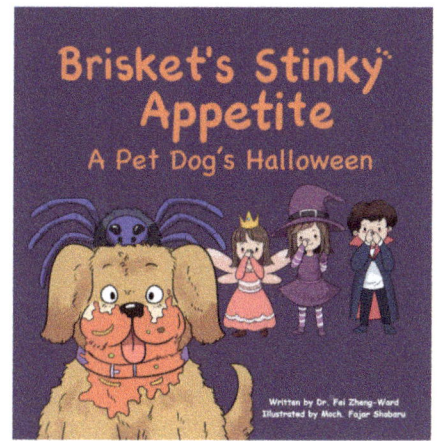
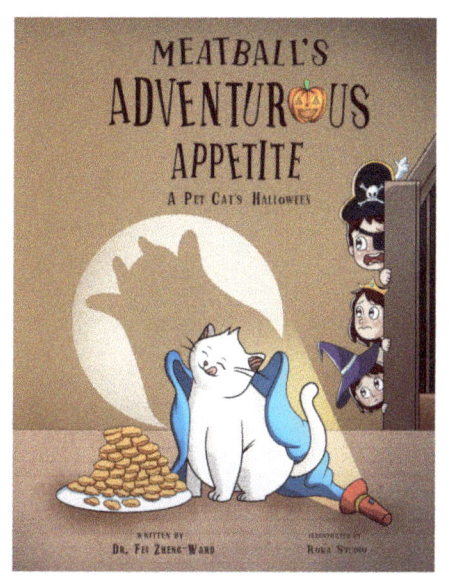
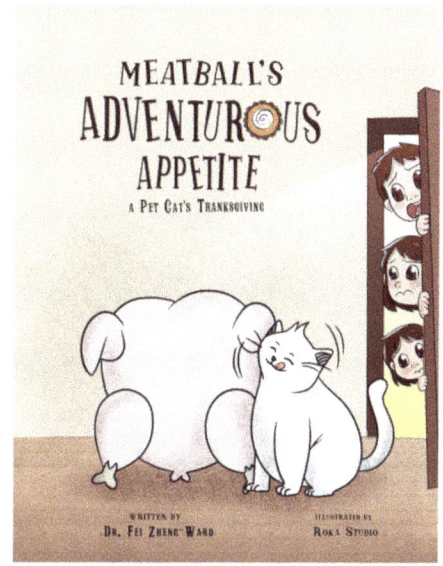
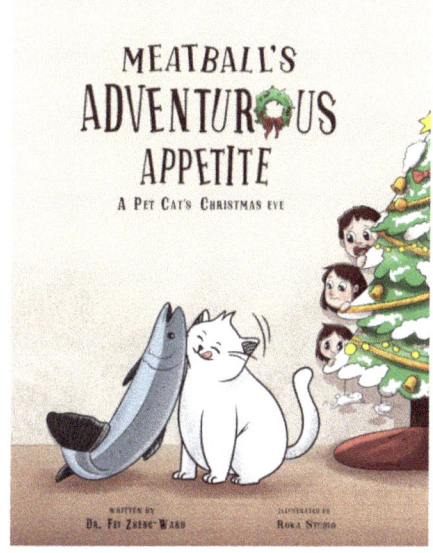
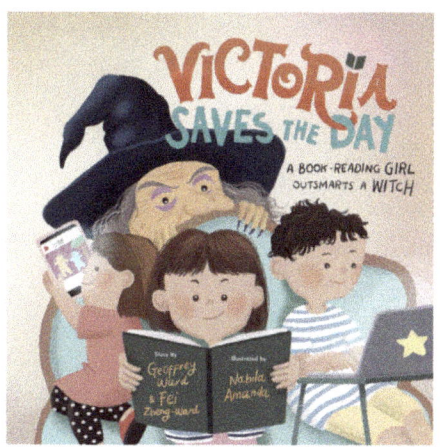
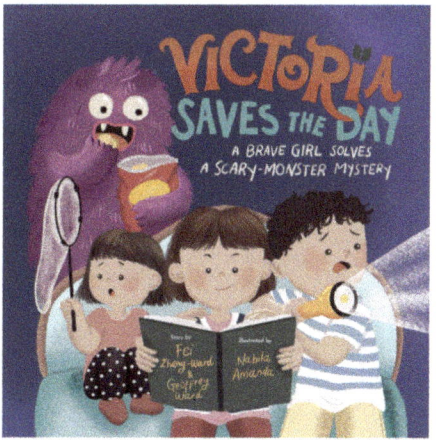
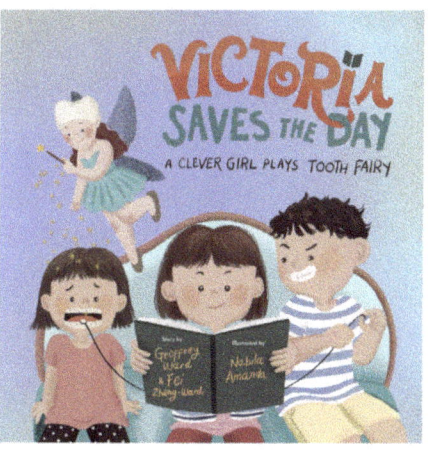

www.ingramcontent.com/pod-product-compliance
Lightning Source LLC
Chambersburg PA
CBHW040000040426
42337CB00032B/5168